LAPAROSCOPY – AN INTERDISCIPLINARY APPROACH

Edited by **Ivo Meinhold-Heerlein**

Laparoscopy – An Interdisciplinary Approach
Edited by Ivo Meinhold-Heerlein

Published by InTech
Janeza Trdine 9, 51000 Rijeka, Croatia

Technical Editor Sonja Mujacic

Cover Designer InTech Design Team

Additional hard copies can be obtained from orders@intechopen.com

Laparoscopy – An Interdisciplinary Approach,
Edited by Ivo Meinhold-Heerlein
p. cm.
ISBN 978-953-307-299-9

For EU product safety concerns:
IN TECH d.o.o., Prolaz Marije Krucifikse Kozulić 3, 51000 Rijeka, Croatia,
info@intechopen.com or visit our website at intechopen.com.

Meet the editor

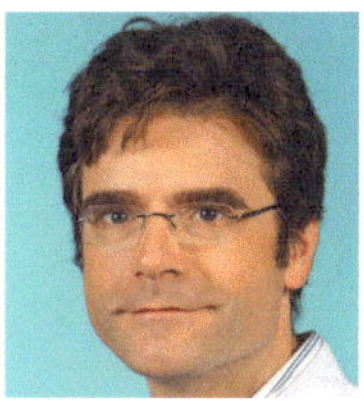

Dr. Meinhold-Heerlein trained at the University of Lübeck and the University of Freiburg and specialized in Obstetrics and Gynaecology at the University of Kiel. He has gained extensive experience in gynaecological endoscopy and oncology both within Germany and abroad. He has been serving as acting head of the Kiel School of Gynaecological Endoscopy and is an internationally recognized authority in endoscopic surgery. He has contributed to teaching and training programmes in Africa, Asia, and Europe. He is currently Assistant Professor and Acting Head of the Department of Gynaecology and Obstetrics at the University Hospital Aachen. He has received numerous scientific awards for his contributions to Gynaecology and Obstetrics within Germany.

Contents

Preface

Many pioneers with different specialties have contributed to the development of operative laparoscopy: It was the urologist Max Nitze (1848-1906) who invented cystoscopy as the very first step of endoscopic surgery. The gastroenterologist and surgeon Georg Kelling (1866-1945) constructed an air insufflation apparatus and performed the first laparoscopy on a dog. The gynaecologist Hans Frangenheim built the first abdominal insufflator and the gynaecologist Kurt Semm (1923-2003) – known as the father of operative gynaecologic endoscopy – performed the first laparoscopic appendectomy.

Today, laparoscopy is widely used by urologists, surgeons, and gynaecologists. Technical advances of recent years have now enabled us to perform most of the open procedures laparoscopically.

The today's spectrum includes benign and cancer surgery in all three disciplines of urology, surgery, and gynaecology, and has led to decreased surgery-conditioned morbidity since laparoscopic surgery – when compared to open surgery – reduces blood loss, postoperative pain, hospital stay and duration of recovery, respectively. It is, therefore, self-evident that a universal textbook of laparoscopy has to cover important procedures of all three disciplines.

Experts of each field have written informative chapters which give practical information about certain procedures, indication of surgery, complications and postoperative outcome. Wherever necessary, the appropriate chapter is illustrated by drawings or photographs.

May this open access book reach many endoscopic surgeons around the globe to enable them to improve their laparoscopic skills, to broaden their spectrum, or just to inspire them about this beneficial technique.

Aachen, July 2011

Ivo Meinhold-Heerlein
Department of Gynaecology and Obstetrics, University Hospital Aachen
Germany

Part 1

Urology

1

Laparoscopy in Urology: An Overview

Richard Zigeuner
Department of Urology, Medical University of Graz, Graz, Austria

1. Introduction

The idea of inspection of the abdominal and other cavities in humans is not and invention recent years but dates back to the early 20th century. However, technical limitations prevented the widespread use of the technique. Along with technical progress laparoscopy became a tool of increasing popularity, but its use was mainly limited to diagnostic inspection of the abdomen for gynaecological and gastroenterological indications. The breakthrough of laparoscopic surgery was the development of laparoscopic cholecystectomy, which within few years was established as the golden standard approach.
In these early days, laparoscopy was still far away from being standard of care in the field of urology. In 1989, the first cases of laparoscopic pelvic lymphadenectomy in prostate cancer patients have been performed and published be Schuessler et al (Schuessler et al., 1991). In the early 1990s, some centres advocated laparoscopic pelvic lymphadenectomy prior to radical prostatectomy or radiotherapy for prostate cancer, since treatment with curative intent was indicated only in cases with histologically negative nodes. Meanwhile along with the development of laparoscopic and robot-assisted prostatectomy, pelvic lymph node dissection if indicated is usually performed together with radical prostatectomy in the same session.
In 1990, the first laparoscopic varicocele repair has been performed, followed by the first laparoscopic nephrectomy performed and published by Clayman and co-workers in 1991 (Clayman et al., 1991). In the pioneer times of laparoscopy, varicocele repair was one of the most frequently used indications to establish this novel technique. However, this indication has been widely abandoned due to more restrictive indications with regard to surgery in varicoceles in general (Diegidio et al., 2011). Moreover, a clear advantage of laparoscopy compared with the small incision of open surgery could not be demonstrated.
Subsequently the laparoscopic approach became increasingly accepted by the urological community. Nephrectomy for primary benign and furthermore also for malignant diseases, via either transperitoneal or retroperitoneal approach, performed with or without morcellation, became more and more accepted. Hand-assisted laparoscopy was developed to facilitate surgery especially during the learning curve in these pioneer days. Indications for the laparoscopic approach were expanded towards cryptorchidism, adrenalectomy, nephroureterectomy, retroperitoneal lymph node dissection for testis cancer, renal cyst decortication, nephropexy, or lymphocele fenestration.
Adrenalectomy for adrenal tumours has been developed in the early days of laparoscopy and has been established and maintained as golden standard approach in adrenal surgery

including phaeochromocytomas except for cancer. The advantage is evident: The adrenal is a small organ but its location requires usually big incisions in open surgery, whereas laparoscopy provides excellent visualization of the adrenal region and in many cases there is no need to extend incisions for specimen retrieval.

Retroperitoneal lymph node dissection in patients with testis cancer has been developed as an alternative to the open approach which requires a median laparotomy from the xyphoid down to the symphysis and frequently leads to retrograde ejaculation in this young patient group. However, retroperitoneal lymph node dissection in general is performed rarely nowadays since the majority of non-metastatic patients undergo risk-adjusted observation, whereas metastatic patients are primarily treated with chemotherapy.

One of the larger steps in advancing laparoscopy was the development of nephrectomy. Meanwhile, the guidelines of the "European Association of Urology" (Ljungberg et al., 2010) suggest the laparoscopic approach as gold standard if tumour nephrectomy for renal cell carcinoma is indicated, whereas the open approach is used only in patients with large tumours, tumour thrombus, enlarged nodes or multiple abdominal operations. In absence of randomized trials, oncological outcomes appear to be identical with the open approach, thus there is no evidence that laparoscopy by itself impacts on prognosis. However, with regard to morbidity and invasiveness, clear advantages in favour of laparoscopy have been reported. Basically, laparoscopic nephrectomy can be performed via trans- or retroperitoneal approach. Comparative studies did not demonstrate differences with regard to perioperative morbidity or oncological outcomes.

Laparoscopic nephroureterectomy for urothelial carcinoma of the upper urinary tract is another indication for laparoscopy in urological malignancies. The main difference is that the entire ureter together with a bladder cuff needs to be resected, which is not required for renal cell carcinoma. The main difficulty in this regard is the handling of the distal ureter, since opening the urinary tract has to be strictly avoided in this type of cancer. Most laparoscopic surgeons therefore perform the nephrectomy laparoscopically, whereas the distal ureter and bladder cuff are removed via a lower abdominal incision required for specimen removal (Zigeuner & Pummer 2008).

Moreover, there is a more frequent indication to perform a lymph node dissection in urothelial cancer compared with renal cell carcinoma which may be difficult in advanced cancers. Consequently, laparoscopy in upper tract urothelial cancer is not yet considered the golden standard approach, although retrospective comparative studies did not demonstrate a detrimental effect of laparoscopy with respect to oncological outcomes. According to current guidelines, laparoscopic nephroureterectomy is reserved for locally confined cancers, whereas the advanced cases should be managed by open surgery.

The development of laparoscopic live donor nephrectomy contributed to an increasing acceptance of live donor nephrectomy on the background of continuously scarcely available kidneys obtained from cadaver donors.

The above mentioned indications have in common that they require mainly ablative techniques. Along with increasing surgical skills and experience, urologists throughout the world developed techniques for more and more complex indications requiring reconstruction of parts of the urinary tract. The most challenging and crucial part of laparoscopic reconstructive procedures is undoubtedly intracorporeal suturing and knotting. Reconstructive surgery includes procedures like ureterocystoneostomy, uretero-ureterostomy, bladder autoaugmentation, pyeloplasty, nephropexy, or bladder neck suspension, each of which has been performed in mostly smaller series. More frequent indications compared to the ones mentioned before include small renal masses, prostate cancer, and bladder cancer. Along with establishing laparoscopic radical prostatectomy and partial nephrectomy, each of these procedures performed either via a transperitoneal or retroperitoneoscopic approach, suturing techniques gained importance as these indications became more and more widely accepted. Indications were expanded towards radical cystectomy and extended pelvic lymph node dissection for muscle-invasive bladder cancer, even with urinary diversions constructed completely intracorporeally.

During the past decade indications for organ sparing surgery (partial nephrectomy) for renal cell carcinoma have undergone significant modifications. Since Robson standardised radical nephrectomy for renal tumours in 1969 this approach remained standard for about 25 years even for small tumours. After slowly increasing acceptance of partial nephrectomy for small (<4cm) renal tumours in the presence of a normal contralateral kidney, the past years brought new insights into possible harmful effects of radical nephrectomy. There is an increasing body of evidence that loss of renal function after nephrectomy increases long term cardiovascular morbidity and mortality, especially if the glomerular filtration rate decreases below 45. Thus, current recommendations suggest to preserve the kidney whenever technically feasible. While there is an expanding indication for partial nephrectomy, the open approach is still considered golden standard for this operation (Ljungberg et al., 2010). However, along with the advances of laparoscopy, laparoscopic partial nephrectomy becomes increasingly accepted. The laparoscopic approach is mainly indicated in smaller, exophytic tumours, whereas the more complex cases are operated by open surgery.

Laparoscopic radical prostatectomy was another progress in the field of laparoscopy. Initially established as a transperitoneal procedure, the extraperitoneal approach was developed subsequently. Although no clear advantage of laparoscopic prostatectomy compared with the open retropubic approach could be demonstrated yet (Ficarra et al., 2009), the procedure has gained popularity and is offered as a standard approach in many centres.

A revolution in laparoscopy was the development of robot-assisted surgery. The technical difficulties due to the inherent limitations of degrees of freedom of rigid laparoscopic instruments contributed to the development of this technique. The major difference of the robot in comparison with conventional laparoscopy is a tremendous improvement in performing complex maneuvers due to articulating instruments. Robot-assisted radical prostatectomy was the first operation to establish this technique. The most challenging step in radical prostatectomy by conventional laparoscopy is the vesicourethral anastomosis, since intracorporeal suturing in the narrow space of the pelvis is technically difficult. Especially this step was facilitated by the robot which enables a wide range of angular movements of the instruments intracorporeally. Although the robotic approach has never been (and presumably will never be) evaluated in prospective controlled trials in comparison with either open surgery or conventional laparoscopy (Ficarra et al., 2009), it is increasingly utilized throughout the world for complex reconstructive procedures.

Consequently, indications for robotic surgery were expanded to other operations requiring any form of intracorporeal reconstructive surgery, like urinary diversion after cystectomy, partial nephrectomy or pyeloplasty.

Most recently, attempts have been initiated to further decrease invasiveness of laparoscopy by development of single incision laparoscopic surgery (SILS), also known as laparoendoscopic single-site surgery (LESS) which uses angulated instruments inserted through one multi-channel trocar (Canes et al., 2008), as well as natural orifice transluminal endoscopic surgery (NOTES) which is preformed via pre-existing orifices like mouth, rectum, or vagina. Whereas SILS is continuously gaining popularity, experience with NOTES in humans is still very limited. Due to the increasing use of robotic surgery, a combined use of these novel techniques (combining robotic assisted surgery with either SILS or NOTES) is increasingly utilised (Rane & Autorino, 2011)

2. Preoperative considerations

2.1 Indications-contraindications

As in any medical treatment or surgical procedure, the key to success is a correct indication. Without any doubt, the first step to indicate any procedure is a precise assessment of patients' history including any previous surgery as well as comorbid conditions. All standardized investigations which are routinely required to be performed prior to any procedure under general anaesthesia apply for laparoscopic surgery exactly the same way. In patients with significant comorbidities, close communication with the anaestesiologists is essential, especially in patients suffering from severe chronic obstructive pulmonary disease, since high intraabdominal pressures resulting from the pneumoperitoneum may result in impaired or even insufficient respiration.

There are a couple of absolute contraindications to laparoscopic surgery. Mainly, infectious conditions in the operative field, like peritonitis or abscess formation represent contraindications, since pressure elevation in a bacterially contaminated environment may result in bacterial dissemination und ultimately septicaemia. Massive haemorrhage in the peritoneal cavity and/or retroperitoneum, either due to trauma or postoperatively, represents another contraindiciation due to impaired visualisation and lack of effective bleeding control mechanisms. Uncorrected haemorrhagic diathesis represents a contraindication as in open surgery as well. However, in case of emergency, when time to correct a coagulopathy is lacking, an open surgical approach will permit haemostasis more effectively (Eichel et al., 2007).

Relative contraindications to the laparoscopic approach include previous abdominal or retroperitoneal surgery, morbid obesity, suspected fibrosis in the operative field due to previous inflammatory or traumatic conditions, excessive ascites, pregnancy, aortic aneurisms, or size of the organ to be operated (e.g., large renal tumours or polycystic kidneys).

Whenever extensive intraperitoneal adhesions have to be expected, entering the peritoneal cavity must be undertaken with maximal care. In this case, open minilaparotomy access with direct vision might preferable over the Verress needle technique. Alternatively, a retroperitoneoscopic approach can be chosen if the patient had undergone previous transperitoneal surgery. The same applies the other way round, if the patient had had open surgical procedures in the retroperitoneum, a transperitoneal laparoscopic approach may be the saver alternative (Eichel et al., 2007).

In morbidly obese patients, technical difficulties may occur from insufficient length of instruments, which may prevent access to the operative field, necessity for higher intraabdominal pressures to ensure adequate visualisation, as well as difficulties in anatomic orientation due to excessive adipose tissue. However, in experienced hands,. obese patients have been shown to benefit even more from the minimally invasive approach with regard to postoperative morbidity compared with normal weight patients (Klingler et al., 2003).

The size of the affected organ, which applies mainly to the kidney from a urological point of view, may be a limitation for the laparoscopic approach. Very large renal tumours, especially if they are located on the upper pole, may restrict the available space required for mobilisation of the specimen in a way that complete specimen mobilisation is made impossible, thus enforcing conversion to open surgery. The same limitation applies for large polycystic kidneys. Pathologically enlarged adjacent organs, like liver or spleen may also limit surgical space and a higher risk of injury to these organs must be taken into consideration in these patients when indicating a laparoscopic approach.

In patients with excessive, yet non-malignant ascites, bowels normally float on the fluid and are consequently at risk for injury when entering the peritoneal cavity. In such cases, comparable to what was noted with regard to previous abdominal surgery, either an open access under direct vision or a retroperitoneal approach should be undertaken. If a transperitoneal procedure is chosen, care must be taken to ensure a watertight closure of the abdominal wall to prevent fistula formation (Eichel et al., 2007).

In case of pregnancy, all efforts must focus on protection of the gravid uterus. As a result of pre-existing compression of the vena cava by the gravid uterus, additional elevation of the intrabdominal pressure may result in hypotension. Moreover, hypercarbia might be detrimental to the fetus and should be avoided. Thus, a pneumoperitoneum of no more than 10mmHg is usually recommended for laparoscopy during pregnancy. Beyond the 20th week of pregnancy the laparoscopic approach is no more feasible in most cases due to working space limitations corresponding with the size of the uterus (Eichel et al., 2007).

In patients with large aortic or iliac aneurysms, a preoperative consultation of a vascular surgeon is mandatory. Care must be taken to avoid vascular injury by trocar placement. Again, entering the peritoneal cavity under direct vision or performing a retroperitoneoscopic procedure should be preferred.

Preoperative imaging is mainly determined by the underlying condition to be operated. Thus, standardized imaging procedures have to be properly performed regardless which surgical approach is chosen. However, in several cases the size or location of a tumour impacts on the decision of the surgical approach, especially in renal masses. The decision whether to perform a radical or partial nephrectomy, via an open, transperitoneal-laparoscopic or retroperitoneoscopic approach is dependent on the findings on preoperative imaging.

2.2 Patient preparation

As for any intervention, a precise informed consent must be obtained prior to surgery. A minimally invasive procedure offers clear advantages for the patients' postoperative course. However, minimal invasiveness does not equal minimal risk of complications. Patients must be informed about the typical risks of the procedure. This includes the possibility of conversion to open surgery, either due to fibrosis, adhesions, bleeding with impaired visualisation or lesions to adjacent organs. The possibilities of bowel injury with the ultimate consequence of bowel resection and even colostomy, the risk of splenectomy or pancreatic lesions for left-sided renal surgery, liver injury for right-sided renal surgery, injury to any of the larger blood vessels, urinary leakage in any procedure opening the urinary tract (like radical prostatectomy, partial nephrectomy, bladder augmentation, pyeloplasty, urinary diversion, ureteral reimplantation), loss of the kidney if partial nephrectomy was indicated or nerve injuries in pelvic or retroperitoneal lymph node dissection need to be discussed. In addition, possible complications associated exclusively with the laparoscopic approach, like hypercarbia, gas embolism, subcutaneous gas emphysema have to be mentioned as well (Eichel et al., 2007).

Prior to surgery, bowel preparation is required if a transperitoneal approach is chosen, since overdistended bowels may limit working space considerably and expose the patient to a higher risk of bowel injury.

Although laparoscopic procedures in general have been reported to be associated with lower blood loss than the corresponding open surgical procedures, significant bleeding cannot entirely be ruled out. Thus, packed red blood cells should be made available prior to the laparoscopic approach as in open surgery, if indicated by the character of the procedure (Eichel et al., 2007).

3. Intraoperative considerations

3.1 Patient positioning

The patients' position is dependent on the intended surgical procedure. For procedures in the retroperitoneum (like any renal or adrenal as well as retroperitoneal lymph node dissection) which are performed via a transperitoneal approach, it is advisable to place the patient in a modified lateral position with a dorsal decline of approximately 30 degrees. This position permits a more supine position for getting access to the abdominal cavity, as it is required for establishing the pneumoperitoneum by Verress needle or open access, whatever is preferred. At the end of surgery, the table can be moved again towards a supine position to facilitate specimen retrieval and wound closure. To perform the intracorporeal steps of the laparoscopic procedure, the table is moved to place the patient in a strictly lateral position. Thus, bowels will move away from the operative field by gravitation and additional trocars are often not necessary. We also omit kidney rests and have abandoned flexing the table in order to increase the distance between ribs and iliac crest as it is indispensable for performing a flank incision in open surgery. In almost all patients the pneumoperitoneum by itself will provide ample space on the patients abdomen to enable adequate trocar placements. Since flexing the patients' spine may cause additional morbidity postoperatively especially in patients affected by spinal disorders, this positioning appears to be advantageous.

If a retroperitoneoscopic approach is preferred, the patient is in a strictly lateral position from the beginning of the operation. In this case, it is necessary to elevate the patients flank by a kidney rest and to flex the table exactly as in a flank incision in open surgery in order to achieve a sufficient distance between the ribs and the iliac crest. From this much more dorsally located position the pneumoretroperitoneum alone will not provide sufficient space for trocar placement.

The decision, whether a transperitoneal or retroperitoneal approach is chosen for renal surgery usually relies on personal experience of the surgeon and a history of abdominal surgery. Currently there is no evidence that the approach by itself impacts on outcomes of the procedure ((Eichel et al., 2007; Desai et al., 2005).

Procedures performed in the pelvis, like radical prostatectomy or cystectomy, require an elevated position of the pelvis (Trendelenburg) to permit the bowels to move away from the operative region, just as described before for renal surgery. The elevation of the pelvis has to be more pronounced if a transperitoneal approach is chosen. For extraperitoneal radical prostatectomy a less pronounced Trendelenburg position is adequate.

3.2 Beginning of the procedure

3.2.1 Transperitoneal approach

Before the laparoscopic procedure can get started, a pneumoperitoneum has to be established. The most commonly used gas for insufflation in laparoscopy is CO_2. The advantage of CO_2 is its excellent solubility in blood which is essential to prevent gas embolism due to high gas pressure in presence of venous leaks. The major disadvantage of CO_2 is the risk of hypercarbia in patients suffering from severe pulmonal disorders. In these patients, helium may be used as insufflant, which, however, is much less soluble in blood than CO_2 and consequently associated with a higher risk of gas embolism. Oxygen, which is well soluble in blood as well is not an adequate insufflant since it leads to intracorporeal combustions and even explosions if fulguration is used (Eichel et al., 2007).

To establish the pneumoperitoneum, two techniques can be used: either a closed approach using a Verress needle, or an open approach.

If the Verress technique is used, the needle is usually inserted at the cranial circumference of the umbilicus with the patient in a supine position. Care must be taken to avoid injury to bowels and major blood vessels during insertion of the needle. In normal weight patients, the needle is usually inserted in direction towards the pelvis to avoid bowel injury, whereas in obese patients insertion is usually done in a more perpendicular fashion. The intended intraabdominal gas pressure is usually set at no more than 15mm Hg. It has been shown that higher pressures are able to to increase the intraabdominal volume only marginally (Mc Dougall et al., 1994).

The Verress technique can also be used if the patient is in a lateral position. In this case, the needle is usually inserted either in the lower abdomen or in a subcostal position. In a lateral position, it is essential to place the needle not in the midline but more laterally, otherwise the insertion is associated with a high risk of bowel injury.

Serveral methods to confirm a correct needle position have been described: using a syringe filled with some saline, an aspiration test can be performed to check whether blood or bowel contents are aspirated. If no aspiration can be seen, saline is injected into the needle. If the needle position is correct in the peritoneum, no resistance will be felt during saline injection. If there is any doubt regarding the correct position, a drop of saline can be placed on the Verress needle. By elevating the abdominal wall, the drop will pass spontaneously into the abdominal cavity, provided that the needle is placed correctly. If the needle is in a correct position, it is possible to advance the needle without resistance. If the tip of the needle is still in a preperitoneal position, gas insufflation will immediately show high pressure and low Flow, pointing to an increased resistance of insufflation.

The possible complications of the Verress technique can be safely avoided by using an open technique. In this case, a slightly larger incision is required to perform a mini-laparotomy. The size of the incision is of minor importance, since it can be used for specimen retrieval at the end of the procedure. A possible disadvantage of the open access is gas leakage, which, however, can be safely avoided by placing a suture incorporating skin and fascia before inserting the trocar. Then, the unloaded trocar is inserted, the suture is tied and the insufflation gets started. While the open access technique has its clear advantages over blind access in patients with previous abdominal surgery, we use the open access technique in all laparoscopic operations at our institution and did not note a single failure or bowel injury so far. The tightening of the incision by suturing can be replaced by using a balloon trocar, which covers the incision from inside the abdominal wall and prevents gas leakage.

Hand-assisted laparoscopy had some popularity in the pioneer days of laparoscopy. Nowadays the hand-assisted technique has been widely abandoned. One still valid indication for hand-assisted laparoscopy is live donor nephrectomy for transplantation. If a hand port is used, a proper incision is made, and after opening the abdominal cavity the port is inserted and the pneumoperitoneum can be established via the hand port.

3.2.2 Extraperitoneal approach

In contrast to intraperitoneal approaches, where ample space is present without additional manipulation, the working space needs to be created artificially for any extraperitoneal approach. For these indications, a small incision is made just enough to permit insertion of the surgeon's index finger. To get access to the kidney, the patient is in a strictly lateral position. The incision is usually made below the tip of the 12th rib in the mid axillary line. After entering the retroperitoneal space, the psoas muscle and the lower pole of the kidney are identified by palpation of the retroperitoneal space Then, in most cases a balloon dilatation of the extraperitoneal space is performed. This dilatation can be performed under direct visual control by using transparent balloons, thus minimising the risk of blind and blunt injury of vital structures. By dilatation the required working space is created between the psoas muscle and the posterior layer of the Gerota's fascia, thus placing the kidney together with its adipose capsule anteriorly. Since the incision is located at the level of the lower pole of the kidney, the balloon is directed cranially to enable a complete mobilisation of the posterior Gerota's fascia and to provide direct access to the renal artery. If additional space is required depending on the procedure, additional dilatation can be made in a caudal direction like for nephroureterectomy or more cranially for partial nephrectomy of upper pole tumours or adrenalectomy, respectively. Only after creation of an adequate working space, placement of the working trocars is possible and safe.

For extraperitoneal radical prostatectomy, similar principles apply with the main difference that the patient is in a supine position with a 30 degrees head-down decline of the table. The first incision is usually made just below the umbilicus, and the balloon is directed caudally towards the pelvis to create a working space preperitoneally.

Basically, the Verress technique can be applied also for extraperitoneal procedures. However, the established tests the prove the correct position of the needle as described for the transperitoneal approach cannot be used outside the peritoneal cavity. Moreover, insufflation alone creates only a small working space, which is usually inadequate for trocar placement. Thus, additional dissection of the retroperitoneum is required. Consequently, most surgeons use the open access technique for retroperitoneal procedures.

3.2.3 Trocar placement

Once pneumoperitoneum or -retroperitoneum have been established, the trocars have to be placed. If a Verress technique had been used for insufflation, the primary trocar for insertion of the laparoscope is place first. If an open access technique had been used, the primary trocar is already in place and the laparoscope can be inserted. Prior to insertion of the laparoscope, the light cord has to be connected and the camera has to be white balanced as in any endoscopic procedure. It is advisable to warm the laparoscope to body temperature to prvent fogging of the lens intracorporeally. After inserting the laparoscope, the operative field is inspected with special focus on intraperitoneal adhesions close to the intended port sites, as well as any other anatomical abnormalities. Additional trocars can be placed under direct vision. Number and size of the required working trocars depend on the procedure and on the diameter of the instruments which have to be passed through the trocar during surgery. Nowadays trocars are routinely equipped with valves enabling the use of 5mm instruments through a 10mm trocar without loss of gas pressure. Basically, two types of trocars regarding the way of entering the abdomen are available: On the one hand, bladed trocars cutting through the abdominal wall and usually equipped with a safety shield that covers the blade after entering the abdomen, on the other hand non-cutting trocars which simply spread the muscle and fascial fibres of the abdominal wall without causing any cutting damage. Consequently, the latter trocars have been shown to cause less bleeding and postoperative hernias (Eichel et al., 2007). Moreover, suturing of the abdominal wall is not required after removal of blunt trocars, whereas closure of the port is mandatory after use of cutting trocars of 10mm or more.

With respect to placement of the trocars care must be taken to avoid injury to underlying sutures and to provide sufficient distance between the trocars. Ideally, the trocar placement corresponds with the operative field which should be located within the borders of the ports sites.

For intraperitoneal procedures, the trocars are placed in a triangular or quadrangular fashion depending on the number of trocars used. If the trocars are located to closely to each other, intracorporeal interference of the instruments is likely. On the other hand, very large distances between the ports may require very wide movements of the surgeons's arms with the result of increased physical efforts for the surgeon and possible problems due to insufficient length of instruments as well as intracorporeal acute angles aggravating adequate preparation. In most cases, a distance of approximately 10-12cm between the trocars appears adequate.

Transilluminating the abdominal wall from inside to chose the correct port site is helpful to avoid injury to larger vessels within the abdominal wall. Skin incisions are made just large enough to permit insertion of the respective trocar, which is then inserted under direct vision. If possible, the trocars should be directed towards the operative field, otherwise moving the instruments may be more difficult. In our experience, any left-sided retroperitoneal procedure can be performed by using just one camera port and 2 working channels. Separate trocars for retraction of bowels or spleen can be omitted in the majority of cases. For right-sided retroperitoneal surgery, one additional 5mm trocar is inserted below the xyphoid to enable retraction of the right lobe of the liver.

For retroperitoneal access to kidney or adrenal gland, trocars are frequently placed in a line parallel to the lower edge of the 12th rib (sites are located at the lateral edge of the erector spinae muscle, below the tip of the 12th rib and anteriorly in the anterior axillary line). Since limited space is available in this region, the patient is positioned in a standard flank position just as in open surgery with elevation of the kidney rest and flexion of the table. The trocars need to be placed close to the 12th rib to enable access to the upper pole of the kidney. If necessary, a fourth trocar can be placed more caudally above the iliac crest for retraction of the kidney.

Extraperitoneal access to the pelvis is mostly used for radical prostatectomy and requires four working channels, which are usually placed in an inverted "U"-shape fashion.

Usually at least one 12mm working channel is required for most procedures to permit passage of endoclip applicators, right angle dissectors, insertion of the specimen retrieval bag, drainage placement or interchanging the insertion site of the laparoscope for

visualization from a different perspective. Whether additional working channels consist of 5mm or 12mm trocars depends on the difficulty of the operation and the surgeon's experience.
Recently, single port devices have been developed which enable insertion of three or four instruments through one multichannel port. Since in this case no distance between the working channels is available, the problem of intracorporeal clashing needs to be overcome by use of curved or flexible instruments which provide adequate angulation inside the body. This method is mainly used for procedures which require some extension of the incision for specimen retrieval, like nephrectomy. The advantage of the single port access is that the incision required for the single port device is sufficient for specimen retrieval in most cases without extension, and additional incisions for working trocars can be spared.

3.3 Performing the procedure

In order to perform and finish a laparoscopic procedure successfully, two major prerequisites must be fulfilled. The first one is to duplicate the principles of open surgery. The second one is excellent visualisation of the operative field. The principles of open surgery depend on the respective procedure to be carried out. It is essential not to agree to any compromise regarding oncological safety. If there is any doubt regarding the feasibility of the laparoscopic approach with respect to oncological outcomes, it is advisable to choose an open approach. It is not acceptable to enforce short term perioperative benefits by all means on the expense of long-term harmful outcomes.
The key to excellent visualisation is high standard camera equipment. Most lenses have a diameter of 10mm and zero or 30 degrees angles. The 30 degree lens has the advantage of varying the perspective in a larger operative field. For preparation of the renal hilar vessels we see an advantage for the 30 degree lens to achieve a better visualisation of the renal artery which is usually located just behind or even slightly cranially to the renal vein. Moreover, dissection of the upper pole and dorsal surface of the kidney via transperitoneal approach is facilitated by the angled lens. In contrast, procedures with a limited space like extraperitoneal prostatectomy are mostly performed using a zero degree lens, since the angled vision is not helpful under these circumstances.
Recent advances include the development of deflectable laparoscopes. Their use, however, is still limited. Three-dimensional systems are mainly used in robotic-assisted procedures (Eichel et al., 2007).
As in open surgery, instruments used for laparoscopy consist of cutting devices like scissors and harmonic scalpels, graspers for retraction, dissectors for blunt preparation, electrosurgical devices using either mono- or bipolar current, clip applicators, vascular staplers, argon beam coagulators and various tissue sealants for haemostasis and needle drivers for suturing. All laparoscopic instruments have in common that they are rotating, thus enabling some variability intracorporeally. None of the instruments used in laparoscopy is distinctly different from those in open surgery. In order to fulfil the prerequisite of duplication open surgery, laparoscopic instruments are simply elongated version of the instruments used in open surgery. With the exception of some clip applicators, stapling devices, and right angle dissectors most of the instruments are available in 5mm diameters.
Whether cutting is performed by scissors together with current or by a (disposable and consequently more costly) harmonic scalpel remains a question of taste. In both cases, some fogging of the operative field will occur leading to impaired visualisation. In this situation

the assistant has to open a valve of one of the trocars to deflate the fog until perfect visualisation is re-established.

As in open surgery, irrigation and suction is sometimes required. Both is performed via one instrument, usually 5mm in diameter, containing an irrigation and a suction unit. If suction is over-used, the pneumoperitoneum will collapse and continuing the procedure will be possible only after re-establishing the proper pressure.

Whereas some titanium clips can be applied via 5mm instruments, the use of polymer clips which provide more security regarding vascular closure is possible only with 10mm instruments. In our own experience, vascular staplers are usually not required when performing a nephrectomy. The renal vein collapses after proper clipping of the artery and can be safely closed with large polymer clips. In contrast to vascular staplers which are disposable instruments the applicators for polymer clips are reusable. As in open surgery, use of electrocautery in close contact to bowels and major vessels has to be strictly avoided to prevent injury to these structures.

In open surgery, retraction of adjacent structures is essential for optimal visualisation of the operative field. The retractors in open surgery are usually large instruments, which cannot be used for laparoscopy. For laparoscopic purposes, as described before, a very important part of visualisation is patient positioning which by itself will replace most of the retractors that would be needed for the same respective operation by an open approach. Several retractors are available. Some of these are inserted in a folded fashion via the trocar and unfolded inside the abdomen like a fan. However, the larger the instrument, the more it may become an obstacle rather than a support for surgery. In our experience, for right sided renal or adrenal surgery we place a 5mm trocar just below the xyphoid an insert a lockable grasper which retracts the right lobe of the liver and is fixed on the peritoneum of the diaphragm just laterally to the liver. Care must be taken to place the trocar as cranially as possible to avoid clashing with working instruments. On the left side, only two trocars are sufficient, no additional retraction is required, if the spleen is mobilised completely from laterally.

The use of tissue sealants is of importance especially when performing a partial nephrectomy. A variety of tissue sealants, fibrin based or non-fibrin based are available. No head-to-head prospective trials comparing the various sealants directly have been conducted. At our institution we use an autologous fibrin glue obtained from patients' own blood at the beginning of surgery (Schips et al., 2006).

Most laparoscopic procedures in urology (with the exception of pyeloplasty, nephropexy, bladder neck suspension, varicocelectomy, ureteral re-implantation) have an ablative character and require retrieval of a surgical specimen. For this purpose, a variety of specimen retrieval bags has been developed. The common principle is that the folded bag is inserted into the patient via a 10mm or 15mm trocar (depending on the size of the specimen and the required bag), then the bag is opened to permit specimen entrapment, followed by closure of the bag enabling intact specimen retrieval. In malignant diseases it is essential to retrieve the specimen within an intact bag to prevent port site metastases (Zigeuner & Pummer 2008). If gas insufflation is applied via the same trocar containing the retrieval bag, it is advisable to insert the insufflation at a different trocar to avoid distension of the organ bag by gas insufflation into the bag instead of the abdomen. If a large specimen is present like in case of nephrectomy, the incision needs to be enlarged until the bag can be removed. For most nephrectomies, skin incisions can be limited to 4-5cm due to elasticity of the tissue, whereas on the level of the fascia consisting of tense and non-elastic connective tissue slightly longer incisions are required dependent on the size of the specimen. For smaller specimens like in partial nephrectomy, prostatectomy or adrenalectomy mostly no or very limited enlargements of the incisions are required.

In the early days of laparoscopy, specimens were routinely morcellated intracorporeally to avoid larger incisions for retrieval. However, in oncological diseases, tissue morcellation may contribute to cancer cell dissemination especially when the bag is damaged by the morcellator. Definitely, even in case of an intact bag, histopathological assessment of the specimen is severely compromised if not impossible. Thus, morcellation has been widely abandoned for oncological diseases.

After retrieval or entrapping of the specimen, the laparoscope is re-inserted to inspect the operative field for bleeding and to perform adequate haemostasis. Lowering the pressure is advisable since smaller venous haemorrhages might be masked by gas pressure. This is especially essential with respect to the venous plexus after radical prostatectomy. A drain is placed if indicated. In most cases of nephrectomy and adrenalectomy drains can be safely omitted. In contrast, any procedure associated with opening the urinary tract and thus amenable for urinary leakage requires drainage. This includes partial nephrectomy, pyeloplasty, nephroureterectomy, radical prostatectomy, cystectomy, ureteral reimplantation, or ureterolithotomy. In case of retroperitoneal lymph node dissection the urinary tract is not opened. However, a typical complication is chylous leakage, which can be easily diagnosed if a drain is in place and is treated dietetically immediately after diagnosis.

Finally the trocars have to be removed. This is done under direct vision to control for bleeding. If cutting trocars have been used, any 10mm or larger port requires closure, whereas 5mm ports do not. If blunt trocars have been used, no suture is required.

Before removing the last trocar, the pneumoperitoneum is deflated. Then, the trocar is removed, the specimen retrieval bag, if still in place is removed after extension of the incision if necessary. Closure of the retrieval incision is performed just as in open surgery.

3.3.1 Intraoperative complications and management:

One complication which is directly associated with laparoscopy and does not occur in open surgery is the risk of hypercarbia resulting from CO_2 insufflation. Since CO_2 is well soluble in blood, it is quickly resorbable from the abdomen an has a low risk of gas embolism. The other side of the medal is that this high solubility in blood may cause hypercarbia. Especially in patients suffering from severe chronic obstructive pulmonary disease (COPD) the high CO_2 levels cannot always be fully compensated by ventilation. Hypercarbia results in increased stimulation of the sympathetic nervous system with the consequence of increased cardiac strain. The risk of hypercarbia is directly related to intraabdominal pressure. The optimal intraabdominal pressure with respect to volume has been described at 15mmHg whereas higher pressures showed only very moderate gain in volume (Mc Dougall et al., 1994). Lowering the pressure to 12mmHg has been shown to reduce cardiac side effects (Eichel et al., 2007).

Other complications exclusively associate with laparoscopy are related to Verress needle insertion. Preperitoneal placement of the needle prevents successful trocar placement. The most important indicator to recognise improper needle positioning is a steep rise in CO_2 pressure associated with a low flow. If the pressure is raised to increase insufflation, an artificial preperitoneal cavity may be created suggesting a correct intraperitoneal needle position. After insertion of the camera, no bowels but only adipose tissue will be visible, and

correct trocar placement will be difficult to obtain. In that case, deflating of this artificial cavity and proceeding with an open access technique is advisable (Eichel et al. 2007).
Vascular injury by placement of the Verress needle is indicated by aspiration of blood into the syringe. Removing the needle without additional manipulations will results in no major bleeding in most cases. However, after establishing the pneumoperitoneum identification and inspection of the punctured vessel is mandatory (Eichel et al., 2007).
Despite excellent solubility of CO_2 in blood, gas embolism cannot be entirely ruled out, especially by incidental unrecognised puncture of a vessel followed by insufflation. This can be prevented by proper check of correct needle placement as described previously. In this case, insufflation must be stopped immediately, followed by hyperventilation with oxygen.
Another possible source of complications is bowel injury, which may be caused by placement of the Verress needle especially in case of intraabdominal adhesions, which may be anticipated by a history of previous abdominal surgery. Puncture of bowels is identified by aspiration of gas and/or bowel contents. If unrecognised, insufflation will lead to asymmetric distension of the abdomen. If bowel puncture is suspected, the needle is removed and either re-inserted at a different site, or the abdomen is entered by open access. After the pneumoperitoneum has been established, identification and inspection of the punctured organ is essential. If no other injury to the bowel except puncture has occurred, usually no further measures are required.
Even after correct needle placement and establishing an adequate pneumoperitoneum, injuries a described before can occur by blind placement of the first trocar. The risk of injury is highest for the underlying bowels. In contrast to needle puncture, trocar induced bowel injury is a much more severe trauma requiring early recognition and repair. Diagnosis is difficult, if the trocar extends through both walls of the bowel. Therefore, after placement of the second trocar it is mandatory to insert the laparoscope through this port to inspect the first blindly placed trocar and ensure proper trocar placement as well as integrity of bowels.
Injury to major vessels, especially aorta or iliac arteries may rarely occur and represents an emergency situation. After blind trocar placement, the diagnosis is made by removing the obturator followed by immediate severe haemorrhage out of the trocar. First, the obturator is reinserted to stop bleeding. Subsequently, immediate laparotomy with vascular repair is required (Eichel et al., 2007).
Most of the complications associated with Verress needle and blind trocar placement can be safely avoided by an open access technique, which is the routinely used approach at our institution. In our own experience, not a single complication was ever noted by open access. However, bowel injury in presence of intraabdominal adhesions may occur even with an open approach. The only disadvantage of the open approach is the need for placing sutures in the fascia to ensure a tight pneumoperitoneum. Suturing on skin level only will allow gas leakage to the subcutis with the consequence of subcutaneous emphysema and hypercarbia. Proper tightening of the abdominal wall may be difficult to obtain especially in obese patients.
After positioning the working trocars under direct vision, bleeding from the port site may occur despite transillumination of the abdominal wall prior to trocar placement. These haemorrhages are usually do not represent an emergency situation, however, proper haemostasis must be ensured. This can be achieved by identification of the bleeding site by using the trocar for compression and followed by electrocoagulation, either from inside the abdomen or from skin level. If the origin of bleeding cannot be identified, placing of haemostatic stitches around the trocar using a perpendicular stitching device which incorporates all layers of the abdominal wall is helpful in most cases.

Any other complications occurring during laparoscopy are typically of surgical origin occurring during the procedure and comparable to those observed in open surgery. The difference lies in the management of the complication resulting from a different approach compared with open surgery. To prevent any injury during laparoscopy, it is essential to ensure adequate visualisation of all instruments during the whole procedure. Any manipulation or even movement of an instrument outside the field of vision may cause damage to adjacent structures. Therefore the camera assistant must be alert to follow all intracorporeal movements of laparoscopic instruments.

The most frequently reported intraoperative complications in laparoscopy are vascular and bowel injuries, followed by injuries to other adjacent structures like liver, spleen, or urinary tract. Bowel injuries may result either from electrosurgical or mechanical tissue damage. Electromechanical damage can occur from direct contact of surgical instruments with bowels and simultaneous activation of coagulation current, or from indirect effects due to insulation failures or contact to other current conducting instruments. Early identification of electrothermic bowel injury is essential for adequate repair. Diagnosis of superficial injuries is made by identification of whitish areas in the serosa. In severe cases the bowel lumen is opened and the mucosa is visible. Dependent on the extent of injury, small serosal lesions may be managed by laparoscopic suturing in skilled hands. If there is any doubt regarding the safety, conversion to an open procedure is advisable. For larger defects, resection of the affected segment followed by anastomosis is required.

To prevent thermal bowel injury, again visualisation of the instruments during any mode of action as well as control of current activation only by the primary surgeon is essential. Moreover, coagulation should only be activated in safe distance to the bowels, which requires adequate visualisation of any endangered structures during the procedure. The camera assistant needs to be instructed to maintain an optimal distance which permits visualisation of the tissue to be fulgurated as well as the structures to be spared from coagulation. Use of bipolar current reduces the risk of electrothermal injury, since indirect effects are minimized, but direct bowel coagulation will result in injury as well.

Mechanical bowel injury can occur by any sharp or blunt instrument. In contrast to thermal lesions, mechanical injuries are usually diagnosed immediately and need to be repaired properly.

Vascular injuries during laparoscopy most frequently occur in renal surgery by injuring renal vein or vena cava. To facilitate venous repair laparoscopically, the gas pressure can be elevated until sufficient visualisation of the defect is possible (Eichel et al., 2007). Subsequent haemostasis is dependent on the location and size of the defect. The available tools include clipping, sealing with any of the commercially available tissue sealants, as well as application of a laparoscopic Satinsky clamp and suturing.

For any arterial bleeding, gas pressure elevation is not helpful since an adequate back-pressure will never be achieved. Arterial injuries that affect non vital vessels can be clipped, if visualised correctly. Injuries to the renal artery might be clipped end ultimately result in a nephrectomy of the affected kidney, even if a partial nephrectomy was intended originally. Injuries of aorta, iliac vessels or superior mesenteric artery will require immediate conversion and consultation of a vascular surgeon.

However, if there is doubt regarding bleeding control by laparoscopy, fast conversion to an open approach is advisable early before the patients becomes haemodynamically unstable. The safest way to perform a fast conversion is elevating two trocars towards the abdominal wall in a fashion that these trocars form a line, followed by incision directed towards the trocars which are in proximate contact with the abdominal wall. Thus, no additional structures are endangered by fast laparotomy except vessels within the abdominal wall which usually can be controlled without troubles.

Ureteral injuries may occur during retroperitoneal or pelvic lymph node dissection, or during partial nephrectomy. If the ureteral injury is incomplete and the continuity of the ureter is intact, transurethral insertion of a ureteral stent combined with continuous indwelling catheter drainage will solve the problem. In case of complete transection of the ureter, end-to end anastomosis or re-implantation, dependent on the site of injury, will be required. Whether this is done laparoscopically or after conversion to an open procedure is mainly a question of surgical skills.

Bladder injury may be repaired by laparoscopic suturing followed by catheter drainage. If suspected, intravesical injection of indigocarmine via the indwelling catheter will help to confirm and identify the lesion.

Splenic injury may occur in left sided renal or adrenal surgery. Smaller lesions can be managed laparoscopically by application of a tissue sealant or by argon beam coagulation, if available. However, in cases of uncontrolled haemorrhage of injury of the splenic hilum, splenectomy performed either laparoscopically or via open approach may be required. For prevention, direct contact of any instruments to the splenic surface should be avoided and the spleen should be safely mobilized away from the operative field. This is facilitated by meticulous dissection of the phrenicosplenic ligaments. If this dissection is extended cranially into the diaphragm, spleen and pancreas can be safely and bluntly dissected from the anterior surface of Gerota's fascia without direct contact to the splenic capsule, and with the patient in a lateral position the spleen will move medially by gravitation without additional retraction, which by itself could cause splenic or pancreatic injury.

4. Postoperative considerations

4.1 Postoperative patient care

One of the major advantages of laparoscopy is minimising postoperative pain, the condition which many patients are more scared of than surgery itself. Due to the minimally invasive character of the procedure, elaborate measures like patients controlled analgesia or peridural catheters are not required in laparoscopy. After day 1 most patients will have adequate pain control by oral analgesics alone. Oral nutrition is usually started the next day. Antibiotics are usually administered as a single shot prophylaxis immediately prior to surgery and do not need to be continued. Prophylaxis against deep venous thrombosis consisting of low molecular heparin and compression stockings is routinely applied like in open surgery.

Indwelling Foley catheters can be removed on day 1 or 2 (with the exceptions of radical prostatectomy and neobladders) dependent on the patients' mobility. Routine laboratory parameters are obtained the same evening and the next morning.

4.2 Postoperative complications

Some postoperative complications originate from surgical injuries that have not been recognised during the procedure.

If thermal injury of the bowels has not been recognised during surgery, symptoms will occur after a delay of several days, with the highest risk on days 3 and 4. Diagnosis of free air intraabdominally is not helpful after laparoscopy in this early phase since it may represent residual gas left after the procedure. Clinical signs and symptoms pointing to ileus and an abdominal CT will aid in diagnosis.

If mechanical bowel injuries are left undiagnosed for any reason, symptoms will develop without the delay that is typical for with thermal injuries. With regard to repair, the same principles apply as described before.

In case of intraoperatively undiagnosed bladder lesions, the patient may develop urinary ascites postoperatively with elevation of serum creatinine due to reabsorption and abdominal symptoms. The diagnosis is made by cystography. As it is standard in traumatology, the management of urinary leakage depends on the location: intraperitoneal lesions require surgery, extraperitoneal lesions may be managed conservatively by indwelling catheter drainage.

If a ureteral lesion had been missed during surgery and is diagnosed postoperatively, signs and symptoms of urinary leakage occur after some days. The diagnosis is confirmed by retrograde ureterography. In the lesion is incomplete, stenting of the ureter is attempted together with catheter drainage. The catheter is removed, after a cystogram shows no extravasation, whereas the ureteral stent is left in place for 6 weeks. In contrast, complete ureteral lesions require again surgical repair together with stenting.

Postoperative pain is usually limited after laparoscopy. A typical pain pattern after laparoscopy is shoulder discomfort. If deflation of the pneumoperitoneum had been incomplete, patients will feel some pain in their shoulder girdle. This is the result of distension of the diaphragm. This sensation is transmitted by the phrenical nerve which originates from the segment C4. Consequently, the sensation radiates to other regions innervated from the same segment.

Any pain exceeding normal values requires evaluation regarding intraoperatively missed injuries as described above or postoperative haemorrhage. Along with clinical evaluation and laboratory parameters focusing on bleeding, inflammation and renal function, an abdominal CT scan will help to clarify the situation. Postoperative chest pain requires exclusion of myocardial infarction and pulmonary embolism just as after open surgery. Specifically for laparoscopy, the frequent shoulder girdle discomfort may mimic pulmonary embolism. Localised pain may result from incisional hernia. If bowel incarceration is suspected, immediate diagnosis by CT is initiated, and after confirmation, surgical repair is required.

Incisional hernias may occur in the later postoperative course as well. Repair can be performed via either a laparoscopic or open approach, dependent on site and symptoms. In case of emergency of an incarcerated hernia, the open approach is preferred. Hernias are more frequently seen after use of cutting trocars of 10mm or more and in the scars of organ retrieval incisions, whereas hernia formation is unlikely in port sites when blunt trocars are used.

After lymphadenectomy, lymphocele formation may occur, especially after extended pelvic lymph node dissection as it is advocated for cystectomy as well as for radical prostatectomy in high risk cases. Due to compression of adjacent structures, edema of lower extremities, thrombosis, hydronephrosis and in case of infection fever may occur. Large lymphoceles can be easily diagnosed by ultrasound and confirmed by CT. First step is decompression by percutaneous drainage, which can be applied either by ultrasonic or CT guidance. Differential diagnosis includes urinoma, which can easily be confirmed or ruled out by measuring creatinine concentration of the drained fluid. Whereas lymph shows serum-equivalent creatinine levels, urine will always show multiple of serum levels. Thus, even the fluid contains a mixture of lymph and urine, even small amounts of urine can be diagnosed reliably.

A special type of lymphocele is chylous fistula, which may occur after left-sided surgery in the upper retroperitoneum, especially after any renal procedure, adrenal surgery, or retroperitoneal lymph node dissection for testis cancer. If a drain had been placed during the procedure, the milky chylous fluid will be visible in the drain as soon as the patient will re-start fat-containing diet. If no drain has been placed, patients return after discharge with increasing abdominal distension and discomfort, since the fatty chylomicrons are not reabsorbed by the peritoneum. For symptomatic relief, a CT-guided drainage may be inserted. The treatment of chylous fistula consists of fat-free diet and usually does not require surgical interventions. In the rare event that chylous fistula does not resolve by dietary measures, surgery is facilitated by preoperative fatty diet which helps to identify the fistula intraoperatively, thus permitting clipping or ligation (Eichel et al., 2007).

5. References

Canes, D.; Desai, M.M.; Aron, M.; Haber, G.P.; Goel, R.K.; Stein, R.J.; Kaouk, J.H.;& Gill, I.S.(2008). Transumbilical single-port surgery: evolution and current status. *European Urology* Vol 54, No. 5 (November 2008), pp. 1020-1029.

Clayman, R.V.; Kavoussi, L.R.; Soper, N.J.; Dierks, S.M.; Meretyk, S.; Darcy, M.D.; Roemer, F.D.; Pingleton, E.D.; Thomson, P.G.; & Long, S.R. (1991). Laparoscopic nephrectomy: initial case report. *Journal of Urology* Vol. 146, No. 2 (August 1991), pp. 278-82.

Desai, M.M.; Strzempkowski, B.; Matin, S.F.; Steinberg, A.P.; Ng, C.; Meraney, A.M.; Kaouk, J.H.; & Gill, I.S. (2005). Prospective randomized comparison of transperitoneal versus retroperitoneal laparoscopic radical nephrectomy. *Journal of Urology* Vol 173, No. 1 (January 2005), pp. 38-41

Diegidio, P.; Jhaveri, J.K.; Ghannam, S.; Pinkhasov, R.; Shabsigh, R.; & Fisch, H.(2011). Review of current varicocelectomy techniques and their outcomes. *British Journal of Urology International.* 2011 (Epub), doi: 10.1111/j.1464-410X.2010.09959.x.

Eichel, L.; McDougall, E. & Clayman, R.V. (2007). Basics of Laparoscopic Urologic Surgery, In: *Campbell-Walsh Urology 9th edition,* (pp. 171-220), Saunders-Elsevier, ISBN 13 978-0-7216-0798-6, Philadelphia, PA, USA

Ficarra, V.; Novara, G.; Artibani, W.; Cestari, A.; Galfano, A.; Graefen, M.; Guazzoni, G.;, Guillonneau, B.; Menon, M.; Montorsi, F.; Pate,l V.; Rassweiler, J.& Van Poppel, H. (2009). Retropubic, laparoscopic, and robot-assisted radical prostatectomy: a systematic review and cumulative analysis of comparative studies. *European Urology* Vol. 55, no.5 (May 2009), pp.1037-1063.

Klingler, H.C.; Remzi, M.; Janetschek, G.; & Marberger, M.(2003). Benefits of laparoscopic renal surgery are more pronounced in patients with a high body mass index. *European Urology* Vol. 43 No. 5 (May 2003) pp. 522-527

Ljungberg, B.; Cowan, N.C.; Hanbury, D.C.; Hora, M.; Kuczyk, M.A.; Merseburger, A.S.; Patard, J.J.; Mulders, P.F.; Sinescu, I.C.; & European Association of Urology Guideline Group (2010). EAU guidelines on renal cell carcinoma: the 2010 update. *European Urology* Vol. 58 No. 3 (September 2010), pp. 398-406.

McDougall, E.M.; Figenshau, R.S.; Clayman, R.V.; Monk, T.G.; & Smith, D.S. (1994). Laparoscopic pneumoperitoneum: impact of body habitus. *Journal of Laparoendoscopic Surgery*, Vol. 4 No. 6 (December 1994), pp. 385-391

Rane, A. & Autorino, R. (2011). Robotic natural orifice translumenal endoscopic surgery and laparoendoscopic single-site surgery: current status. *Current Opinions in Urology* Vol. 21, No.1 (January 2011) pp. 71-77.

Schips, L.; Dalpiaz, O.; Cestari, A; Lipsky, K.; Gidaro, S.; Zigeuner, R.; & Petritsch P (2006). Autologous fibrin glue using the Vivostat system for hemostasis in laparoscopic partial nephrectomy. *European Urology*, Vol. 50 No. 4 (October 2006) pp. 801-805

Schuessler, W.W.; Vancaillie, T.G.; Reich, H. & Griffith, D.P. (1991). Transperitoneal endosurgical lymphadenectomy in patients with localized prostate cancer. *Journal of Urology*, Vol. 145, No.5 (May 1991), pp. 988-91

Zigeuner, R. & Pummer, K. (2008). Urothelial carcinoma of the upper urinary tract: surgical approach and prognostic factors. *European Urology* 2008 Vol. 53 No. 4 (April 2008), pp.720-731.

2

Laparoscopic Radical Prostatectomy

Pierluigi Bove and Valerio Iacovelli
Tor Vergata University of Rome, Rome
Italy

1. Introduction

Cancer cure, normal continence and preserving sexual function are the primary goals of radical prostatectomy (RP). By adopting the laparoscopic technique with adherence to established oncological principles, the aim is to duplicate the open surgical method in its entirety.

1.1 Historical aspects

Laparoscopic radical prostatectomy (LRP) has become an established treatment for organ-confined prostate cancer and is increasingly performed at selected centers worldwide even though open radical retropubic prostatectomy (RRP) is widely considered the treatment of choice (Walsh, 2000).

For the first time in 1992, Schuessler, a non-academic, attempted the first LRP assisted by two endourologists with laparoscopic experience in renal surgery (Schuessler et al., 1992). These pioneers were able to successfully perform 9 LRP procedures, but found no benefit over open prostatectomy. The operation was cumbersome and difficult with unacceptably prolonged operative time. The authors concluded that the procedure offered no advantage compared to RRP (Schuessler et al., 1997).

In 1998 Guillonneau et al. detailed their stepwise approach to transperitoneal LRP. After substantially improving the techniques at Montsouris in France, Guillonneau and associates published their series demonstrating substantial improvements in postoperative convalescence. The operation was shown to be feasible, but more importantly, although the learning curve remained steep (Guillonneau et al., 1999).

Since then, various European teams have added to the overall experience with this technique (Bollens et al., 2001; Rassweiler et al., 2001; Türk et al., 2001; De La Rosette et al., 2002). In USA, even experienced laparoscopists remained very skeptical about LRP. Gill and Zippe, who at that time focused on renal laparoscopic surgery, were one of the few who established a program of laparoscopic pelvic surgery (Gill & Zippe,2001).

After 1997 LRP has slowly risen in popularity and became, in some centers, the surgical approach of choice for the treatment of the localized prostate cancer for its advantages. The lower blood loss and transfusion rate associated with the laparoscopic approach together with shorter hospital stay, reduced catheterization time, better pain control and the faster return to everyday activities seem the most encouraging improvements obtained (Hoznek et al., 2005).

2. Preoperative assessment: Patient selection

2.1 Indications

The indications for LRP are identical to that for open surgery, that is, patients with clinically localized prostate cancer (stages T1 and T2) with no evidence of metastasis either clinically or radiographically (CT, Computer Tomography and bone scan), a low PSA level (<10 ng/mL), a Gleason score < 7 and are age 70 or younger (Steinberg & Gill, 2004).

2.2 Contraindications

As with open surgery, previous abdominal and/or perineal surgery (such as transurethral resection of the prostate, pelvic surgery, laparoscopic inguinal hernia repair), history of radiation to the prostate, morbid obesity, large prostate size (e.g., >100g) and/or androgen deprivation may complicate organ dissection and are more challenging, but these features are not by themselves contraindications for laparoscopic prostatectomy.
Specific and absolute contraindications to minimally invasive laparoscopic prostatectomy include an active peritoneal inflammatory process, an uncorrectable bleeding diatheses or the inability to undergo general anesthesia due to severe cardiopulmonary compromise, akin to open surgery (Brown et al., 2005).

3. Preoperative preparation

3.1 Bowel preparation and prophylaxis

No bowel preparation is given usually. Since operations are done under general anesthesia, patients should receive nothing by mouth for at least six hours before surgery. Fasting starts at midnight before surgery. Thromboprophylaxis is implemented with good hydration, placement of compressive elastic stockings on the lower extremities, and low-molecular-weight heparin. A single intravenous dose of a 3rd generation cephalosporin low molecular weight subcutaneous heparin are given on call to the operating room. Patients admitted the day before surgery receive 4000 units of low molecular weight heparin the night before surgery (e.g., Enoxaparin such as Clexane®, 40 mg sc 1 × day) and continued daily until the patient is discharged from the hospital. Blood type and crossmatch are determined (Rosenblatt et al., 2008) .

3.2 Informed consent

The importance of informed consent is due to patient information. Patients undergoing LRP must be aware of the potential for conversion to open surgery, for possible bleeding, transfusion and infection. Impotence, incontinence, incisional hernia as complications and the risks of general anesthesia must also be presented to the patient.

3.3 Operating room personnel and configuration

Skills and training are key requirements of the operating room staff. The surgical team includes a scrub nurse, circulating nurse and surgical assistant(s). Only one surgeon is usually sufficient, but a second assistant may be useful in retracting tissues. The scrub nurse must be very versed in the laparoscopic surgery field in order to accomplish this procedure.
The surgeon operates from the patient's left side, and the first assistant is placed at the opposite side of the surgeon. The laparoscopic cart is placed at the patient's feet, while the instruments table and the coagulation unit are positioned at the left side of the patient. The

scrub nurse is positioned beside the left lower extremity of the patient. The video monitor is placed between the patient's feet, at the eye level of the surgeon. (Fig. 1).

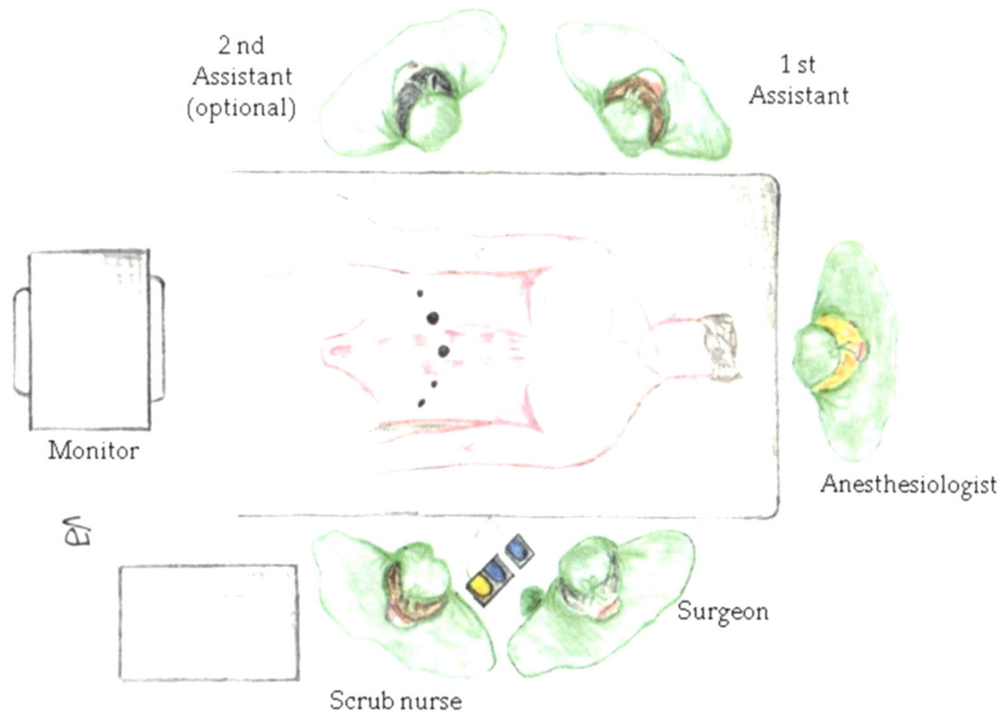

Fig. 1. Operating room personnel, position of the operative team and trocar configuration for laparoscopic radical prostatectomy. Steps are placed in front of the surgeon, and the bipolar and monopolar pedals are placed over the steps.

3.4 Instruments

It is preferable to choose the best instruments, even if they are more expensive. A good instrument is more effective and lasts longer. The following list corresponds to our personal preferences and does not claim to be exhaustive (Vallancien et al., 2002).

The following list corresponds to the essential instruments used for laparoscopic prostatectomy:

- An 18 Fr Foley catheter;
- 3 reusable, long 5-mm trocars, including 1 with an insufflators;
- 2 reusable 10-/12-mm trocars;
- 3 long forceps;
- 1 pair of unipolar forceps;
- 2 large bipolar forceps;
- A small bipolar forceps;
- 2 needle holders;
- Pledgets;
- 1 metal Béniqué sound;

- 1 rectal bougie;
- 1 aspirator-irrigator;
- Suture materials: they must be solid and must not form loops spontaneously;
- Lactomer 9-1: 3/0, 5/8 or 3/8 needle;
- Polyglactin 910: 2/0, 36 needle for the retropubic space;
- Polyglactin 910 1/0, 40 needle for the abdominal wall;
- Video equipment adapted to urology;
- Video camera and monitor with excellent definition;
- A rapid insufflators with modern safety features.

3.5 Patient positioning

The patient is positioned supine. The legs are slightly abducted and are fixed into the padded receptacles. The arms are fixed beside the body in arm padding. The abdomen is prepared from the xiphisternum to the perineum, including the genitals. The patient is secured to the table with adhesive tape, with both arms alongside his body. The thighs and the lower extremities are also secured. Strapping must be secure enough to prevent patient movement with the 30–40°. Trendelenburg position is used during surgery, but breathing should not be impeded. The base of the table must be positioned below the patient's hip to avoid elevation of the abdomen while in the Trendelenburg position.
Foam pads are used to pad the patient at all bony prominences to minimize pressure injury. A 18Ch Foley urethral catheter with 10mL in the balloon is introduced after the placement of the sterile drapes. An orogastric tube is placed to decompress the stomach. The abdomen, pelvis, and genitalia are skin prepared in case conversion to an open procedure is required.

3.6 Anesthesia considerations

General anesthesia is required in LRP. Before patient positioning is necessary to establish an accurate pulse oximetry, intravenous access and blood pressure gauge placement. Special attention is paid to the control of the CO_2 insufflation and pneumoperitoneum consequences such as oliguria and hypercapnia. Prompt and continues adjustments by the anesthesiologist and surgeon may be required.
Absolute contraindications: history of intracranial surgery or intracranial tumors. Relative contraindications: respiratory failure, severe heart failure and glaucoma.

4. Surgical technique

Comprehensive understanding of the anatomical landmarks and its implications in the patient's future quality of life are mandatory when attempting the procedure. The normal anatomical landmarks to consider during trocar placement while performing any of the minimally invasive techniques are umbilicus, anterior superior iliac spine, pubic symphysis and lateral border of rectus sheath. Generally, these procedures are accomplished using 4 to 6 trocars placed in a "W" or *inverted fan* configuration. Vesicourethral anastomosis is accomplished by either a continuous or an interrupted suturing technique, and the prostate is usually removed via an extension of the umbilical port site.
Several approaches to minimally invasive prostatectomy have been described, including the transperitoneal (TP) or Montsouris 1 and extraperitoneal (EP) or Montsouris 2. Each approach has its own unique merits and drawbacks. Each operator must choose the preferred technique based on experience (Levinson & Su, 2007; Vallancien et al., 2002).

The extraperitoneal approach provides a rapid access to the space of Retzius, minimizes bowel complications and intra-abdominal organ damage. The extraperitoneal method closely resembles the open RRP. However, the pelvic and prostate anatomy is magnified during laparoscopy, making dissection of important structures much more precise. Because no bowel is manipulated, the chance of an ileus or injury is decreased. Less Trendelenburg positioning is needed since the bowel does not need to be retracted, which may result in improved anesthetic and cardiovascular factors. Intraperitoneal contamination is not a concern, and the confined retroperitoneal space may aid in venous tamponade. The main limitation is the restricted working space, but with experience this does not seem to be an important drawback. However, recent studies comparing transperitoneal versus extraperitoneal approaches have not found any significant differences (Brown et al., 2005; Cathelineau et al., 2004). The extraperitoneal approach may be preferable in obese patients as it may shorten the distance between the trocar insertion site and operative field, and in patients with previous abdominal surgery where time-consuming adhesiolysis is avoided and the risk of bowel injury is minimized (Rassweiler et al., 2006).
We prefer to adopt the extraperitoneal route. Steps are placed for the surgeon, and the bipolar and monopolar pedals are placed over the step.

4.1 Extraperitoneal approach

The various steps of the operation are:

1. Abdominal access, insufflation and port placement
2. Dissection of the retropubic space
3. Opening of the pelvic fascia on each side
4. Mobilization of the bladder
5. Dissection of the seminal vesicles
6. Dissection of the neurovascular bundles
7. Haemostasis of vessels of the retropubic space
8. Dissection of the apex and section of the urethra
9. Vesicourethral anastomosis
10. Extraction of the surgical specimen and closure of the abdomen wall.

4.1.1 Abdominal access, insufflation and port placement

The first extraperitoneal laparoscopic approach was described in 1997 by Raboy et al. (Raboy et al., 1997). With this approach, the initial step is to create the extraperitoneal space. Five laparoscopic ports are used: two 10-/12-mm ports and three 5-mm ports. A 1,5 cm cutaneous incision is made at 1 cm below the inferior margin of the umbilicus. . With blunt finger dissection, a space is created anterior to the peritoneum. The subcutaneous fatty tissue is dissected with blunt scissors, resulting in visualization of the superficial fascia (rectus sheath). The fascia is grasped by two Kocher clamps and incised (Fig.2).
The first trocar is inserted into the abdominal wall without preliminary insufflations. The instrument must be directed more tangentially than for the transperitoneal route (20° to the horizontal instead of 45°). A trocar-mounted balloon dilator device is inserted into the preperitoneal space and about 300 ml of air is inflated to develop the space of Retzius as shown in Fig.3 (pneumo-Retzius). Pneumodissection occurs spontaneously. The scope is introduced and is used to collapse the loose connective tissue in order to enlarge the prevescical space. The pubic arch is rapidly identified and the tissues are largely dissected

on both sides to provide sufficient space. Pneumoextraperitoneum is created (15 mmHg) and four secondary ports are placed in a fan array. This way, secondary trocars are then placed under laparoscopic view by placing them slightly lower towards the pubis, as the working space is slightly narrower than transperitoneal approach. In the *inverted fan* configuration, the second 10-/12-mm port is inserted at the lateral border of the right rectus abdominis muscle to place the bipolar grasper. The three 5-mm trocars are one pararectus on the right iliac fossa and two are place halfway between the anterior-superior iliac crest and pararectus trocars on the left iliac fossa. With port placement in the *fan* configuration, the surgeon operates through the two ports on the left side and the assistant uses the two right-sided ports (Fig.2). (Landman et al., 2004).

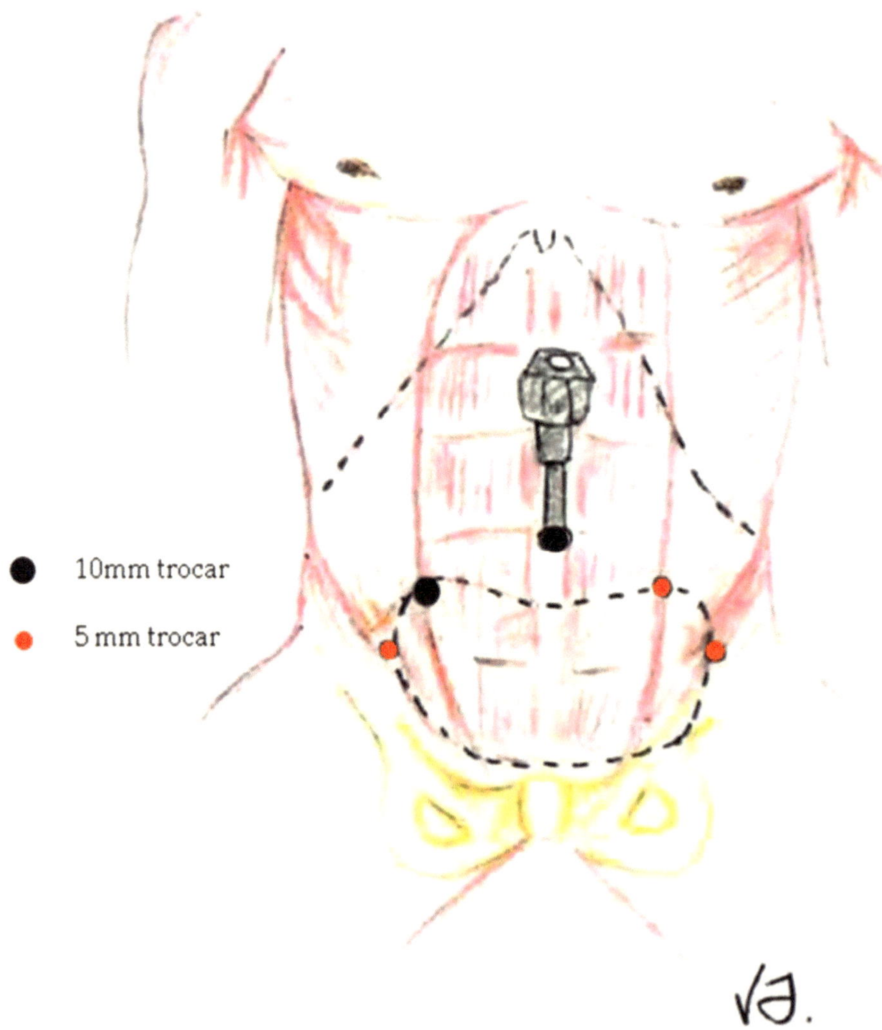

Fig. 2. Access and port placement.

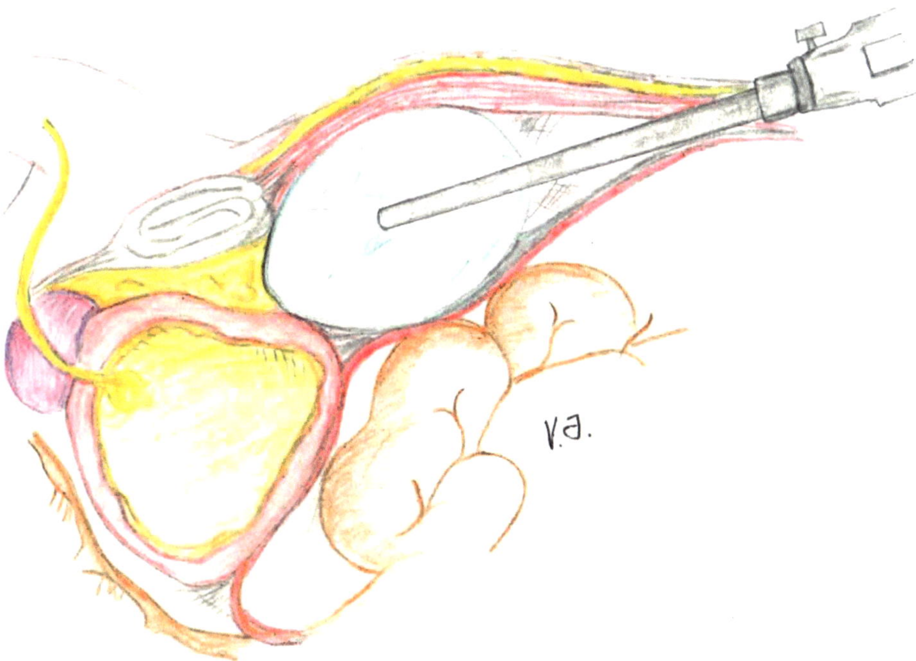

Fig. 3. Trocar-mounted balloon dilator device creating the pneumo-Retzius, a working space for extraperitoneal laparoscopic radical prostatectomy.

4.1.2 Dissection of the retropubic space

The patient is placed in the Trendelenburg position, with the head tilted down approximately $30\text{-}40^{0}$. This position aids the correct displacement of the intestine above the promontory by gently pushing back the loops of the small bowel.

The retropubic space is dissected by simple insufflation after directly placing the 10 mm trocar in an infraumbilical position. This space is rich in fatty tissue. The fibroareolar and fatty tissue layers between the superolateral aspect of the bladder and the medial aspect of the external iliac vein are bilaterally released (Rosenblatt et al., 2008). Once entry into the retropubic space is gained, dissection in the prevesical space of Retzius is performed in a deliberate manner, maintaining hemostasis at all times. The superficial dorsal vein, included in the small fatty area in the midline in the vicinity of the puboprostatic ligaments, is coagulated with bipolar electrocautery. Subsequently, the endopelvic fascia is cleaned bilaterally. The removal of this fatty tissue facilitates visualization and dissection of the bladder neck, which is usually located under the crossing of the fibers of the puboprostatic ligament (Vallancien et al., 2002).

4.1.3 Opening of the pelvic fascia on each side

The pelvic fascia is incised on each side, which partially mobilized the prostate. The right and the left sides of the endopelvic fascia are incised along the dotted line. The prostate is

retracted contralateral placing the endopelvic fascia on stretch. The endopelvic fascia is incised using a J-hook electrocautery or cold endoshears. The fascial incision is carried distally up to the lateral-most puboprostatic ligament. The fibers should not be divided close to the prostate to avoid lacerating the large veins that cross lateroposterior to the prostate (Kelly's veins). As the two layers of endopelvic fascia become more adherent moving toward the apex, they are then incised with the monopolar scissors to open the plane between the prostate and the endopelvic fascia. Visualization of the prostate apex is the endpoint of this dissection.
The completed incision of the endopelvic fascia bilaterally, exposing the convex contours of the prostatic lobes. The apex of the prostate is defined bilaterally. (Fig.4). The lateral puboprostatic ligaments are divided as necessary (Vallancien et al., 2002).

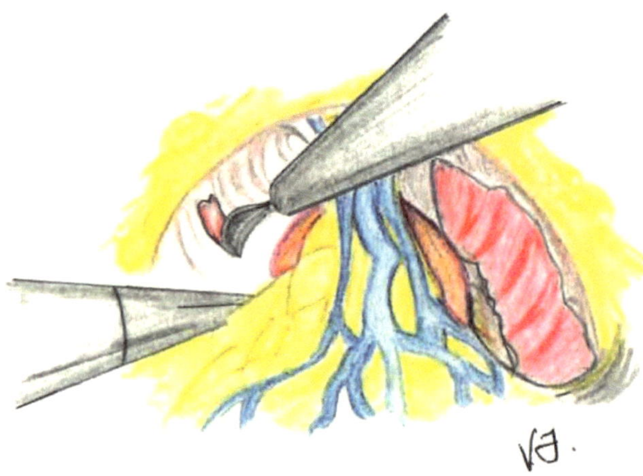

Fig. 4. The fatty tissue from the pubic symphysis is removed espousing the endopelvic fascia and the puboprostatic ligaments. The endopelvic fascia is incised.

4.1.4 Mobilization of the bladder

The bladder neck is situated under the crossing of the fibers of the puboprostatic ligaments. The bladder catheter balloon is inflated with 15-20 ml and is pulled on by the scrub nurse in order to reveal the bladder and its limits with the prostate. The limit between the two organs is most clearly defined by the perivesical fat. The assistant grasps the bladder dome and draws it downwards to give a good curvature. The bladder is incised at its junction with the prostate.
The incision progresses to assume an inverted U-shape to avoid dissecting through the lateral sides of the prostate. At the medial portion of the dissection, the longitudinal muscle fibers of the anterior urethral wall are exposed. The urethra is dissected at its anterior and lateral aspect and then transversally transected (Rosenblatt et al., 2008).
At this point, the Foley catheter is removed and replaced by a Béniqué sound, providing a good visualization of the bladder. The anterior surface of the prostate and the first detrusor muscle fibres are clearly visible. The dissection is carried out from the lateral side to the center and continues to the other side to fully separate the bladder neck from the base of the prostate. This is an important step in order to ensure good preservation of the bladder neck.

As this fase of the operation can cause bleeding, the tissues must be regularly coagulated. One of the best methods of coagulation is bipolar forceps.
Once the bladder is extensively dissected on both sides, it appears to be attached only by the bladder neck around the midline Béniqué sound. The bladder neck is meticulously opened close to the prostate and the urine is aspirated. A tip is to avoid tearing the bladder neck in order to preserve a small diameter. The posterior surface of the bladder neck can be seen. Care must be taken not to perforate the bladder at this level as the ureteral orifices are in close proximity. When the bladder neck is preserved, the ureteric orifices are situated further away. The posterior lip of the bladder neck is grasped with forceps and lowered to provide access to the interprostatorectal plane (Vallancien et al., 2002) (Fig.4).

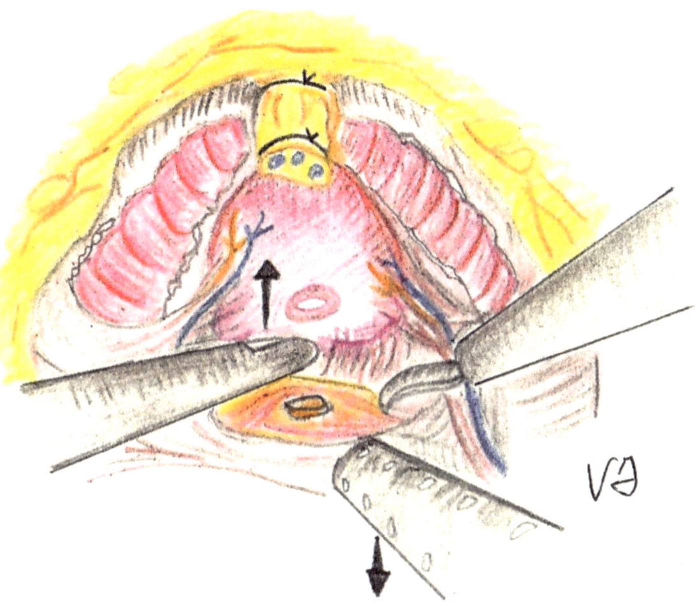

Fig. 1. Bladder incision at its junction with the prostate. Dorsal vein complex appears to be ligated just to focus on the incision. This procedure is done and analyzed later.

4.1.5 Dissection of the seminal vesicles and vasa deferentes

The plane of longitudinal muscle fibers behind the bladder neck is transversally incised to expose the vas deferens. The vertical fibers of the anterior plane of Denonvillier's fascia covering the seminal vesicles are incised (Rosenblatt et al., 2008). The ampullae of the left and right vasa deferentes (or vasa deferentia) can be seen in a fairly midline position, protecting the rectum from damage by the instruments. The ampullae of the right vas deferens is sectioned after coagulation with cold scissors or clipped with a Hem-o-lock clip and divided at its lower point, as in the transperitoneal technique. A large grip is used to simultaneously coagulate the anterior deferential artery. The seminal vesicle is dissected circumferentially from the base to the apex, taking care to control the vessels. It is important to remain flush with its lateral surface to avoid any diffusion of heat and any trauma to branches of the pudendal nerve. The lateral pedicle of the seminal vesicle is dissected and coagulated, and following the inferior pedicle dissection and coagulation, the seminal vesicle tip is then freed. This way, the right vas deferens and seminal vesicle have been completely mobilized. The left vas deferens is dissected in the same way. The left seminal

vesicle is then closely dissected to allow maximum mobilization. The seminal vesicles may then be dissected after the bladder neck dissection is complete, via an anterior approach.
At this time, we preferred to use harmonic or bipolar scalpel in order to avoid dissipation of thermal energy that could damage the nervi erigentes. It is essential to remain close to the seminal vesicles in order to prevent damage to the neurovascular bundles (NVB) and for this reason use of thermal energy should be limited to avoid the neuropraxia of the cavernous nerves, which lie in close proximity to the seminal vesicle. In order to preserve the NVB hemoclips are applied along the lateral aspect and tip of the seminal vesicle to secure the vascular pedicle.
By lifting both vasa deferentia and the seminal vesicles with a grasper, the Denonvillier's fascia is exposed as shown in Fig. 5 (Vallancien et al., 2002).

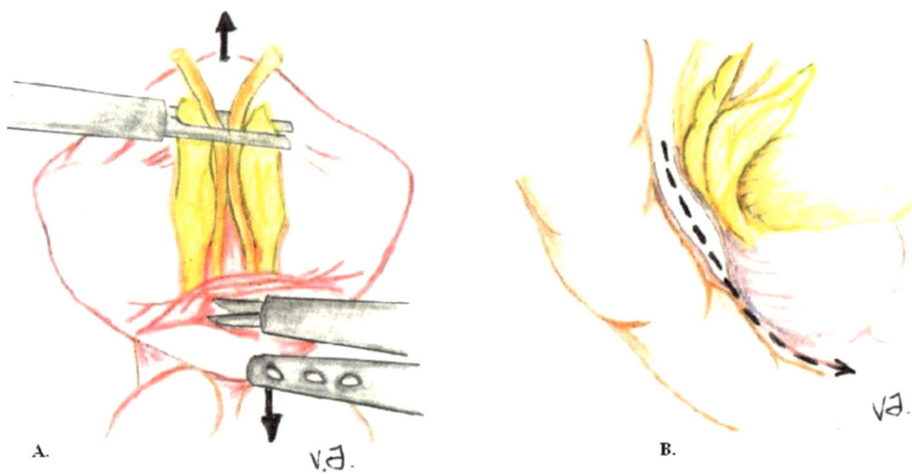

Fig. 5. Dissection of the prostate. A) By lifting both vasa deferentia and the seminal vesicles with a grasper, the Denonvillier's fascia is exposed. A traverse incision is made in Denonvillier's fascia below the seminal vesicles and blunt dissection is used to develop a plane between Denonvillier's fascia and the rectum. B) Dissection towards the prostate apex.

4.1.6 Dissection of the neurovascular bundles

The fibers of the Denonvillier's fascia are stretched and identified when the assistant holds the completely dissected seminal vesicles anteriorly. Two planes of dissection are correct: a) plane between the Denonvilliers' fascia and the prostate, which is the plane developed for neurovascular bundle preservation; b) posterior plane between the rectum and the Denonvillier's fascia—developed in cases of wide excision of the prostate without neurovascular bundle preservation (Rosenblatt et al., 2008).
The Denonvillier's fascia is transversely incised for 2-3 mm in the midline about 0,5 cm below the base of the seminal vesicles that are grasped with forceps and are drawn superiorly placing tension. Blunt dissection is carried out between the Denonvillier's fascia and the rectum till to visualize perirectal fat and the posterior aspect of the prostate.
The seminal vesicles are used to draw on the prostate to start dissection of the right NVB. The assistant inserts forceps into the dissection between the bladder and the prostate. The aspirator is used to lower the bladder to tighten the vescicoprostatic pedicles. Bipolar forceps are used to dissect and ensure haemostasis of the right vesicoprostatic pedicles.

These pedicles can bleed abundantly and good preventive coagulation is essential. The largest vessels visible, should be coagulated separately. The left vesicoprostatic space is opened by drawing the left seminal vesicle towards the right with forceps. Haemostasis is performed in the same way as on the right side with bipolar forceps. The left NVB is situated much lower. At this point, the bladder is completely mobilized. The prostate is only attached by the puboprostatic ligaments and NVBs.

Dissection of NVBs starts with the assistant who holds the forceps placed on the vesicoprostatic dissection and gently retracts the tissues of the NVB with the aspirator. The operator uses bipolar forceps and scissors. Access to the NVB is achieved by dissecting the endoprostatic fascia high on the right lobe to avoid damage to small nerve branches. As the neurovascular bundle usually runs at a minimal distance from the prostate at the level of the apex, the dissection of the bundle is easier at this level. The lobe has a characteristic white color. Dissection is continued along the lobe by gently retracting the NVB with the aspirator. If the capsule is penetrated, the operator must immediately return to the right plane. The prostatic fascia is gradually separated from the lobe, limiting coagulation to a minimum. This phase is only slightly hemorrhagic. Small bipolar forceps are used, advancing step by step to avoid penetrating the prostatic capsule. The NVB is gently drawn towards the right with the aspirator meanwhile the dissected right edge of the prostate is clearly visible. Dissection is continued with scissors and coagulation should be used as little as possible and only using the small bipolar forceps with a reduced power. The right NVB, identified by its arterial pulsations, is dissected, without going as far as the apex. Dissection is terminated in retrograde fashion after having released the apex. On the left side the steps are identical. On both sides dissection must start at the top of the prostate and the lateral part is gradually dissected (Fig. 6 A & B).

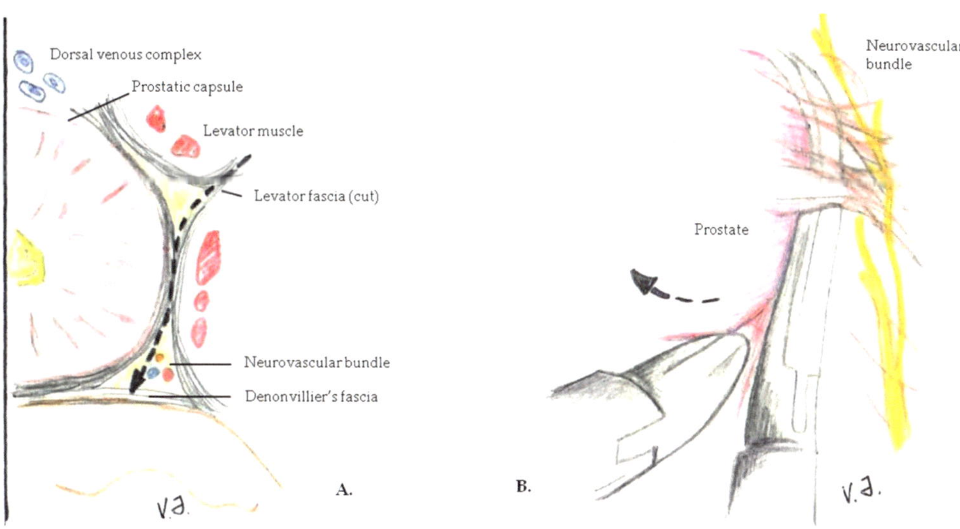

Fig. 6. Dissection of the neurovascular bundles. A) Emi-cross section of the prostate demonstrating the periprostatic fascial planes with respect to the location of the neurovascular bundles. The dashed line indicates the direction of interfascial dissection. B) developing the interfascial plane of dissection. A fine-tipped curved or right-angled dissector in gently passed immediately beneath the levator fascia to develop the interfascial plane of dissection.

The prostate can be stripped on the left. The NVB is perfectly visible. In patients with a history of endoscopic resection, prostatitis or hormonal therapy, the plane of cleavage may be difficult to find.

A simple veil of tissue remains, which is gently retracted. Haemostasis of visible perforating arteries is performed with small bipolar forceps. The prostate has been released and is now only attached by the apex, which will facilitate the following step of ligation of the vessels of the retropubic space, as it becomes very mobile in the lesser pelvis. The two puboprostatic ligaments are preserved. During dissection of the apex and section of the urethra, the operator must continually verify the position of the NVBs in relation to the instruments.

In the case of a very large tumor on one side or if the Gleason score is greater than 7, it is preferable not to perform intrafascial dissection, but to leave one or two millimeters of periprostatic tissue all along the lobe to avoid an excessively high positive margin rate without necessarily resectioning the NVB (Vallancien et al., 2002).

4.1.7 Haemostasis of vessels of the retropubic space

The dorsal vein complex at the apex of the prostate is legated with Polyglactin 910 2/0 suture material on a 36 needle. The needle is introduced through the right medial iliac 10-/12-mm trocar with a n. 10 reducer. There is no clearly defined limit beyond which the needle may be too deep. The Béniqué sound is useful to detect when the needle is inserted too deeply towards the urethra.

At the midpoint of insertion of the suture, push the right needle holder downwards and to the left so that the needle tends to rise upwards towards the left. When this maneuver is not performed, the needle will enter the pelvic muscles on the left side, where it cannot be reached. The needle is grasped on the left side with the right needle holder and is then pulled with the left needle holder, in a harmonious curve to avoid tearing the tissues. The aspirator, held by the assistant in the right medial 5-mm trocar, is used to retract the left prostatic lobe so that the needle remains visible.

As a safety measure, a double suture is performed by inserting the needle more superficially from right to left to ensure excellent haemostasis (Fig.7). The needle is grasped on the left near the puboprostatic ligament.

The suture is tied with four knots. The tissues are coagulated with bipolar forceps (Vallancien et al., 2002).

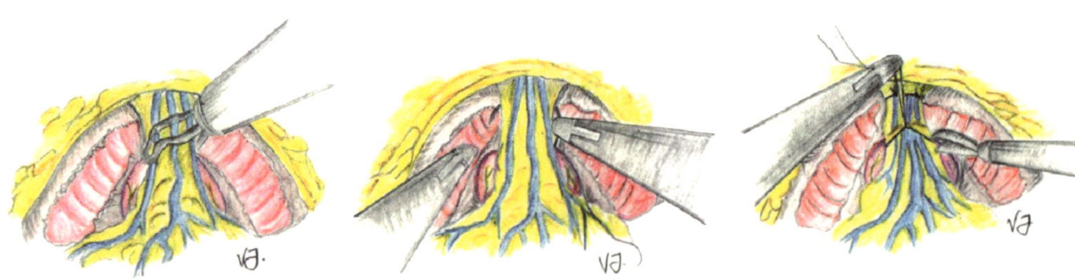

Fig. 7. Dorsal vein complex ligation. The common trunk of the Santorini deep venous plexus and lateral venous plexuses are covered and concealed by the prostatic and endopelvic fascia. Any laceration of these friable structures can lead to considerable blood loss.

4.1.8 Dissection of the apex and section of the urethra

Dissection of the apex starts with retraction of the preprostatic tissues using unipolar scissors. The urethra is reached gradually by incising the frequently thickened tissues covering the anterior surface of the urethra.

Scissors, concave upwards, are used to detach the prostatic apex from preurethral tissues. The Béniqué sound is advanced to make the urethra more prominent. Scissors, concave downwards, are used to retract the apex in order to preserve a maximum of urethra which is incised laterally, avoiding any risk of damage to the left NVB. The same procedure is performed on the right. The posterior surface of the urethra is sectioned at the end. Fibers of the rectourethralis muscle are sectioned, revealing the plane of the rectum. The fibers still attached to the left prostatic lobe are sectioned close to the prostate to avoid damage to the NVB at first on the left and then on the right side. Excessive tension must not be applied to the prostate to prevent rectal injuries. In case of adhesions due to history of prostatitis, multiple biopsies, previous irradiation placing the left index finger in the rectum (finger-assisted laparoscopy) is a practical way to limit the risk of injuries (Vallancien et al., 2002).

4.1.9 Vesicourethral anastomosis

Good-quality needle holders are essential during this procedure. The grip must be powerful and needle holders must be sufficiently long and rigid. The vesicourethral anastomosis requires also an excellent dexterity in the use of needle holders and, especially for a right-hander, the ability to use either the left and the right hand. The suture material must have different qualities such as resistance, no spontaneous loops forming and recognizable colour. During initial experience, the urethrovesical anastomosis is the most time-consuming and challenging part of the operation. However, with experience, suturing is predictable and precise.

Prior to performing urethrovesical anastomosis, bladder neck reconstruction (necessary in only 10–15% of cases) can be performed by placing two to four running stitches posteriorly or anteriorly in a tennis racket fashion. It is important to visualize the position of the ureteral orifices before the closure is initiated to avoid inadvertent passage of the suture through the ureter. The bladder neck is narrowed to approximate the diameter of the urethra (Rosenblatt et al., 2008).

The initial stitch is placed at the 6-o'clock position of the bladder neck and the urethral stump with Lactomer 9-1 3/0 on a 5/8 needle using interrupted suture placed in the same way for all patients. At least three to four needle passes are necessary in a clockwise direction to create an adequate posterior plate.

The first stitch is made from inside to outside on the urethra. The right needle holder is used with a twisted forehand movement (Fig. 8). The needle is passed through the aperture of the Béniqué sound, then introduced into the urethra at 6-o'clock, as the operator gradually withdraws the Béniqué sound with the left hand. The needle is brought out posteriorly near the rectum using the left needle holder, making sure that it has not included the right NVB. The suture must remain strictly in the midline. Movements of needle holders must describe curves to avoid tearing the urethra. The length of suture material is calculated by the length of the 10-/12-mm trocar plus 2 cm. the solidity of this first stitch is verified by pulling on the two ends of the suture, which reveals the urethral lumen. Two sets of forceps are used to grasp the bladder neck, with the mobile jaws facing downwards to enter the posterior lip of the bladder neck. The needle is passed thought the bladder, taking care not to include a ureteric orifice by remaining strictly in the midline at 6-o'clock. The bladder is then lowered

towards the urethra. The knot is composed of four loop, the first two of which are formed in the same direction to allow the suture material to slide freely.
The second suture is performed in a similar way: using the Béniqué sound, the needle is passed with the right hand from inside to outside the urethra at 8-o'clock. Once again, in order to be well coordinated, the maneuver must be performed by the operator himself. The operator holds the needle holder in his right hand and the Béniqué sound in his left hand and gradually withdraws it as the needle holder advances into the urethra. The left border of the bladder sometimes needs to be retracted with the aspirator in order to see the needle leave the urethra. These two bridge suture are essential as they ensure the solidity of the posterior plane of the vesicourethral anastomosis. Sutures are cut 5mm from the knots. Both ends of the knots must be cut before extracting the needle to avoid tearing the urethra. The needle must always be removed through the right medial iliac 10 mm trocar by holding the tip of the needle with the right needle holder, otherwise the needle may be trapped at the entry of the trocar and fall into the abdomen from where it will be difficult and time consuming to find.
The third suture is performed to the right of the first suture at 4-o'clock. The needle held in the right needle holder is inserted into the bladder with a forehand movement from outside to inside and the needle is then extracted with the left hand. The needle is kept in the left hand and is inserted into the urethra from inside to outside. The curve mad by the left hand with the needle holder can be more accurately guided with the right hand. To facilitate passage of the needle using the left needle holder, the urethra is retracted with the Béniqué sound directed towards the left to open the urethra. By simply rotating the left wrist, the needle enters the urethra atraumatically. The needle is extracted with the right needle holder.
The fourth suture is performed to the left. The needle enters the urethra at 9-o'clock over the Béniqué sound, using the right needle holder, with the needle back to front. The left NVB must be clearly visualized to avoid injury. The suture passes from inside to outside the urethra. After extracting the needle with the left needle holder, it is inserted into the bladder from outside to inside, making sure that the left ureteric orifice is not included. The knot is tied inside with 4 loops. The tension on the two ends of the suture held by the needle holders must be equal to avoid tearing the urethra.
The fifth suture is performed to the right from outside to inside, passing first thought the urethra, at 3-o'clock. The position of the needle is unusual: instead of holding the needle, as for the other suture, about 2/3 from the base, the needle is held by the middle with the right needle holder at an angle of about 120°. The needle holder is placed outside the urethra, to the right, and is passed thought the urethra horizontally; the Béniqué sound drawn towards the left opens the urethral lumen. The needle is brought out in the urethra and grasped with the left needle holder to complete the curve without tearing the urethra. The needle is then grasped with the left needle holder and inserted into the bladder, from inside to outside, and is then extracted with the right needle holder. Both hands must be used to accompany the passage of the needles without forcing, to avoid tearing the tissues.
The sixth suture is performed on the left, starting from the urethra, starting at 10-o'clock with the needle held by the right needle holder, with the needle tip facing upwards and towards the right. By simply rotating the wrist, the needle enters the urethra to the left. The needle is recovered with the left needle holder. The bladder is then included from outside to inside before tying the knot inside the anastomosis.

The seventh suture is situated anteriorly and enters the urethra from outside to inside at 11-o'clock. The needle is then taken with the right hand and inserted into the bladder from inside to outside. The knot is tied outside the anastomosis.
The eighth suture starts in the bladder on the right. The needle is inserted from outside to inside, using the right needle holder. The needle is then taken with the left needle holder and enters the urethra immediately, at 2-o'clock, from inside to outside. The knot is tied outside the anastomosis.
The other sutures (9-12) run from the urethra to the bladder anteriorly or from the bladder to the urethra independently. The knots are tied outside the anastomosis. If there is a step between the bladder and the urethra, sutures are added from the bladder to the anterior surface of the bladder. This tennis racket reconstruction is easier to perform than a posterior reconstruction at the beginning of creation of the anastomosis.
Before tying the last anterior suture, the Béniqué sound is removed and the bladder catheter is inserted, making sure that it follows the right passage. If the anastomosis has been correctly performed posteriorly, the bladder catheter rarely passes underneath the bladder. The presence of bubbles from the bladder catheter indicates a false passage and the catheter must be replaced using an angled stylet. After completing the vesicourethral anastomosis, the Foley catheter balloon is inflated with 10 ml. The watertightness of the suture is checked by injecting 250 ml of saline without pulling on the Foley (traction on the balloon could mask a leak) (Vallancien et al., 2002).

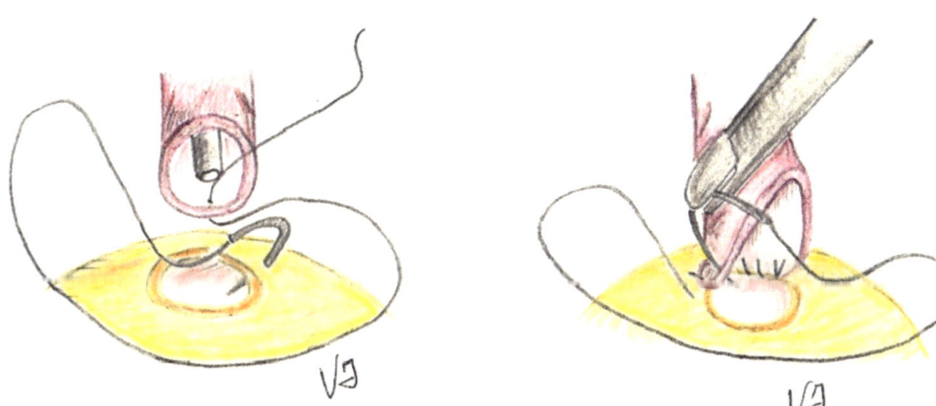

Fig. 8. Vesicourethral anastomosis. The vesicourethral anastomosis requires an excellent dexterity in the use of needle holders and, especially for a right-hander, the ability to use either the left and the right hand.

4.1.10 Extraction of the surgical specimen and closure of the abdomen wall.

Once the vesicourethral anastomosis has been completed, an 8 F suction drain is introduced via the left lateral iliac trocar and is then immediately sutured to the skin after removing the 5-mm trocar. The drain is placed in the pouch of Douglas, which is the most dependent site. It is usually removed on Day 2.
The prostate localized in the right iliac fossa is grasped with forceps inserted via the left medial iliac trocar and transferred to the lesser pelvis where it is placed in an endobag and extracted via the umbilical port.

The scope is therefore transferred to the right medial 10-/12- mm trocar, leaving the umbilical 10-/12-mm trocar free. The umbilical 10-/12-mm trocar orifice is slightly enlarged to allow extraction of the prostate in its bag. The bag is grasped with Kelly forceps and extracted by applying traction and rotation movements. The abdominal wall must be closed meticulously to avoid an incisional hernia. The two angle sutures are inserted before completing the suture by one or two sutures in the midline. Polyglactin 910 1/0 suture material is usually used on a 40 needle (Vallancien et al., 2002).

4.2 Transperitoneal approach

The various steps of the operation are the same as in extraperitoneal prostatectomy, but they are performed in a different order:

1. Patient positioning, insufflation and insertion of trocars
2. Pelvic lymph node dissection
3. Dissection of seminal vesicles and the interprostatorectal space
4. Dissection of the bladder and lobes of the prostate
5. Opening and mobilization of the bladder
6. Dissection of neurovascular bundles
7. Haemostasis of vessels of retropubic space
8. Dissection of the apex and the section of the urethra
9. Vesicourethral anastomosis
10. Extraction of the prostate and closure of the incision.

The Montsouris technique 1 was described by Guillonneau and Vallancien, in which dissection commences initially at the rectovesical cul-de-sac. The sigmoid colon is retracted cephalad and a transverse peritoneotomy created at the second (distal) peritoneal fold in the rectovesical cul-de-sac.

The seminal vesicles and vas deferens are mobilized circumferentially using bipolar cautery. Denonvilliers' fascia is opened to enter the pre-rectal plane. Subsequently the bladder is dropped posteriorly, the space of Retzius developed, the dorsal vein ligated, the bladder neck transected, and the prostatic pedicles incised while preserving the neurovascular bundle if indicated. The urethra is transected, prostate excision completed and the vesico-urethral anastomosis made (Steinberg & Gill, 2004).

The potential advantages of the transperitoneal laparoscopic radical prostatectomy compared to the extraperitoneal approach are a greater working space and reduced tension on the urethrovesical anastomosis. Furthermore, when performing extended pelvic lymphadenectomy for high-risk prostate cancer patients, the transperitoneal technique is technically less demanding than the extraperitoneal approach (Guillonneau & Rozet, 2002; Türk et al., 2001; Vallancien et al., 2002).

5. Postoperative considerations

The nasogastric tube is removed at the end of the procedure. The patient is given appropriate analgesia as per protocol, including intravenous paracetamol during the first 24 h and major analgesics as necessary. The intravenous perfusion is stopped on day 1 after surgery, oral fluids are started the morning after surgery, and a light diet can generally be resumed on day 2. The suprapubic drain is usually removed after 48–72 h or after secretions are below 50 mL. The bladder catheter is removed on day 5 after surgery if urine is clear, but in case of persistent residual haematuria, a cystogram is performed. Normal activity is resumed four weeks after surgery (Rosenblatt et al., 2008).

6. Intra- and perioperative complications

6.1 Operating time

Lengthy operating times have often been reported for laparoscopic radical prostatectomy. However, times have been shown to decrease with experience. Guillonneau and colleagues reported times of 4.6 hours in their first 50 cases, 4 hours in the next 50, and 3.4 hours in the last 140 cases (Guillonneau & Rozet, 2002).
Currently, our average time ranges from 2 hours to 3 hours.

6.2 Intraoperative blood loss, transfusion rates

High intraoperative blood loss and transfusion rates are common problems of prostate surgery. Reports of open prostatectomy series have reported blood loss of 500 mL, 1 L, or more. During laparoscopy, excellent visualization of the dorsal venous complex and a tamponade effect from the 15-mm Hg pressure of the carbon dioxide pneumoperitoneum minimizes blood loss. The necessity of transfusion varied from 1.6% to 31% among the analyzed series (Bove et al., 2009).

6.3 Conversion to open surgery and other perioperative complications

The rate of conversion from laparoscopic to open surgery remains low (0 to 5%), but some centers had a high conversion rate in their early experience. The low conversion rates in all major series are a testimony to the careful introduction of LRP. With increasing experience, even challenging situations, such as cases following previous laparoscopic hernioplasty can be managed (Bove et al., 2009).
Following the current literature we could deduce that there is a 4% (1-6.1%) of intraoperative complications (rectal injury 1.5% (1-2.4%), ileal or sigmoid injury 1% (0.8-1.9%), epigastric vessels injury 0.27% (0-0.5%), bladder injury 0.81% (0-1.6%), ureteral injury 0.36% (0-0.7%), external iliac vein injury 0.09% (0-0.8%). The early postoperative complications amounted to 20.7% of cases and they mainly included anastomotic leakage (10.3%), hemorrhagic complications (2.8%), urinary retentions (2.35%) and ileus (1.4%). However, anastomotic stricture, phlebitis/embolism/thrombosis, urinary tract infections, neurological complications, fistulas, lymphorrea, trocar hernia accounted for percentages below 1% (Bove et al., 2009). These data are summarized in Table1.

Intra and Postoperative Complications	Percentage
Rectal injury	3,3
Ileus/sub-ileus	2,5
Blood transfusion	2,2
Neurologic lesion	1,8
Bowel injury	0,9
Thrombosis/embolism	0,8
Bladder injury	0,4
Renal failure	0,3
Ureteral injury	0,1
Other	0,6
Total complication rate	12,9

Table 1. Main intra and postoperative complications of laparoscopic radical prostatectomy in late series (Lein et al., 2006).

7. Oncological outcome

7.1 Surgical pathology

Prostate cancer is a multifocal disease with an average of seven distinct cancerous sites within each radical prostatectomy specimen. Any surgical procedure aimed at eradicating prostate cancer must completely remove the prostate gland. Then, the removed prostate tissue must undergo pathologic analysis to determine if the edges of the removed tissue (ie, the "surgical margin") show evidence of tumor cells or not (Humphreys et al., 2004).

7.2 Surgical margins and cancer control

Generally, a surgical margin is considered positive if tumor cells reach the "inked" boundaries of the prostate specimen on pathologic examination. The risk of cancer recurrence increases significantly with positive surgical margins independent of pathologic grade, PSA, and DNA ploidy for organ-confined disease. Several series have stressed the importance of surgical margin status in the development of postoperative multivariate models to determine patient prognosis ((Bove et al., 2009; Humphreys et al., 2004).

In the most representative series of laparoscopic radical prostatectomy follow-up is not long enough to give a definitive oncologic evaluation of its surgical efficacy. Nevertheless, preliminary data suggest that this approach can guarantee the same results in terms of cancer control as those of open procedures.

No cases of trocar track metastasis or local relapse have so far been reported after LRP. The extraperitoneal approach avoids this potential risk of intraperitoneal dissemination of tumor cells.

Depending on the surgical approach the location of surgical positive margins differs: the apex with the retropubic radical prostatectomy, the bladder neck with the perineal radical prostatectomy, the posterolateral regions of the prostate (that contain the neurovascular bundles and prostatic pedicles) in the LRP (probably because of the instrument axis and its smaller amplitude during dissection of the prostatic pedicles, which are closer to the trocar ports).

As concerns oncologic results of RP, these are evaluated based on the rate of positive surgical margins (that reflect the quality of tumor excision) and survival with no biological progression.

The positive surgical margins, defined as the presence of cancer at the inked margin of resection on the prostatectomy specimen, influence the prognosis, as they determine a higher risk of biochemical, local and systemic progression.

Authors	pT2	pT3	Overall Positive Surgical Margin Rate
Guillonneau et al. (1000 pts)	15.5%	31%	19.2%
Rassweiler et al. (500 pts)	7.4%	31.8%	19%
Stolzenburg et al. (700 pts)	10.8%	31.2%	19.8%

Table 2. Cancer control: positive surgical margin rate.

The results on the positive surgical margin rate are summarized in Table 2. Recent data, suggest a significant decrease of positive surgical margins over time without any evidence of downward stage migration, in both organ-confined and non-organ-confined disease (Bove et al., 2009).
Given the fact that LRP has only been regularly performed since 1998, information about long term follow-up is unavailable. Although the data continue to mature for LRP series, the short-term biochemical-free recurrence results appear similar to those reported in open radical prostatectomy experience with a biochemical recurrence-free probability between 83 and 94.5% at 3 years as shown in Table 3 (Bove et al., 2009).
Declaring "cure" of prostate cancer requires long-term follow-up. Currently available data are still quite immature. Long-term results on biochemical recurrence-free survival are eagerly awaited.

Authors	3-year Biochemical Recurrence-Free Probability	5-year Biochemical Recurrence-Free Probability	Definition of Progression
Montsouris	90.5%		PSA > 0.1 ng/mL confirmed by a second increase
Heilbronn	83%	73.1%	2 PSA values > 0.2 ng/mL
Johns Hopkins	94.5%		2 PSA values > 0.2 ng/mL

Table 3. Progression free (Montsouris refers to Guillonneau et al., 2002; Heilbronn refers to Rassweiler et al., 2001; Johns Hopkins refers to Pavlovich et al, 2008).

8. Functional outcome

8.1 Continence

The issue of continence is a central concern among most patients. The wide range of incontinence rates reported in the literature indicates the difficulty to obtain an accurate assessment of urinary control after radical prostatectomy. Moreover, the lack of a uniform definition of post-operative continence is crucial to this problem. While some studies use a strict definition of continence as a "no pads" condition, others allow the use of 1 precautionary pad per day as determined by patient report (Bove et al., 2009).
LRP seems initially to offer an earlier continence recovery, but the number of continent patients at one year follow up is comparable to that after open radical prostatectomy. In incontinent patients, even the severity of incontinence seems to be similar after the two procedures. Published reports on the rate of urinary continence after radical prostatectomy (RP) vary widely, at 31–92%, and have been shown to depend on the surgeon's experience, surgical technique (nerve-sparing, bladder neck reconstruction), patient age and, perhaps most significantly, methods of analysis. The physician-determined urinary status after RP can underestimate the problems compared with the results of direct patient-questionnaire surveys (Bove et al., 2009).

Meticulous handling and tissue dissection have allowed the continence rates to improve. Recently Rocco et al. demonstrated that a posterior reconstruction of the rhabdosphincter allowed a rapid recovery of the continence after transperitoneal videolaparoscopic radical prostatectomy.
They report that the musculo-fascial plate, comprised of the striated sphincter, Denonvillier's' fascia, and the dorsal aspect of the prostate, acts as a suspensory system for the prostato-membranous urethra and that its division during RP results in the loss of the posterior cranial insertion of the sphincter, the caudal displacement of the sphincteric complex, and a prolapse of the perineum. Therefore, they propose to reconstruct this musculo-fascial plate by joining the posterior median raphe with the connected dorsal wall of the RS to the residuum of the Denonvillier's fascia and to suspend it to the posterior wall of the bladder, 1-2 cm cranially and dorsally to the new bladder neck (Rocco et al., 2007).

8.2 Potency

Laparoscopic nerve sparing prostatectomy is performed by dissecting the pedicles in an antegrade fashion. This maneuver releases the neurovascular bundle laterally and allows the dissection of the prostate. The delicate NVB is intimately related to the postero-lateral surface of the prostate. As such, complete avoidance of any thermal or electrical energy during lateral pedicle transection and NVB release comprises a hallmark principle during open surgery. However, the use of conventional dissection with hemostatic suture ligatures did not compromise the erectile response to nerve stimulation. Current laparoscopic and robotic techniques for lateral pedicle transection fall short in this important regard, typically using either monopolar or bipolar electrocautery, or ultrasound energy with the harmonic scalpel, with or without clips.
Once postoperative potency is established patients reported ability to achieve sexual intercourse with or without the use of PDE-inhibitors. Potency rates after bilateral nerve sparing LRP have been reported from 33% to 67% in various series worldwide. Most experts agree that at least 18 months of follow-up is necessary to assess potency outcomes adequately (Curto et al., 2006).

Series	Number of BNS	% of Postoperative Potency with or without PDE5-I
Guillonneau et al., 2003	47	66%
Rassweiler et al., 2003	41	67%
Curto et al., 2006	137	58.5%

Table 4. Potency rates (with or without use of PDE5-I) after bilateral nerve sparing (BNS) procedure for patients preoperatively potent.

9. Learning curve: The importance of the mentor

Laparoscopic radical prostatectomy is presently being performed by selected surgical teams with advanced laparoscopic skills. The learning curve is long and steep. Since the surgical technique has now been established, the learning curve should become shorter. Furthermore, as urologists at several centers become proficient at the surgery, colleagues and residents will be trained at the procedure. This can be achieved by an experienced surgeon assisting a novice surgeon.

A learning curve includes the necessity for continuous self-evaluation in terms of cancer control, continence and potency. Many different methods can be used to acquire the technique: dry lab, animal live lab, cadaveric laparoscopic dissection or mentoring with an expert. All of these steps may not be essential, as laparoscopic radical prostatectomy is not too dissimilar to open prostatectomy. The transfer of technology and surgical experience/aptitude is problematic. It has been clearly shown that weekend training courses and weekend laboratory sessions do not translate into clinical ability to perform these procedures. The transfer of training from open surgical experience to newly introduced laparoscopic skills does not occur, emphasizing the need for intensive training (Bove et al., 2009).

These common difficulties clearly highlight the importance of mentoring programs. The mentor is an expert in laparoscopic technique able to direct trainee operative maneuvers increasing his efficiency. Lack of progression is often cited as the most common reason for open conversion during a laparoscopic procedure; in this case the mentor ensures forward progression. The most difficult aspects of this procedure, such as suturing the dorsal vein complex and urethrovesical anastomosis, bladder neck dissection and dissection off of the rectum cannot be effectively learned through laboratory simulation.

We can conclude that an intensive, mentor initiated approach can decrease the learning curve and maintain outcomes (Bove et al., 2009).

10. Cost comparison of LRP versus open radical prostatectomy

Despite the advantages of LRP regarding its minimally invasive character, the operative times for this procedure have been consistently longer than those of retropubic radical prostatectomy and the cost of the disposable operating room equipment is greater, suggesting that LRP is more expensive than RRP. Given the large number of men diagnosed with prostate cancer and presumably seeking treatment, it is desirable that treatment options are not only efficacious but also cost effective (Bove et al., 2009; Humphreys et al., 2004).

11. Conclusions

LRP can be safely performed with early results comparable to open surgery. However, the procedure requires advanced laparoscopic skills and has a steep learning curve. Decreased blood loss during surgery and possibly a shorter duration of convalescence following surgery are definite advantages to the laparoscopic approach. Intracorporeal suturing skills may be developed and refined in the pelvic trainer, to help decrease operating time during early experience.

12. References

Bollens, R., Vanden Bossche, M., Roumeguere, T., Damoun, A., Ekane, S. & Hoffmann, P. (2001). Extraperitoneal laparoscopic radical prostatectomy. Results after 50 cases. *Eur Urol*. 40, 2001, pp. 65-69.

Bove, P., Asimakopoulos, A.D., Kim, F.J. & Vespasiani, G. (2009). Laparoscopic Radical Prostatectomy: a Review. *Int Braz J Urol*., 35, April 2009, pp. 125-139.

Brown, J.A., Rodin, D., Lee, B. & Dahl, D.M. (2005). Transperitoneal versus extraperitoneal approach to laparoscopic radical prostatectomy: an assessment of 156 cases. *Urology*. 65, 2005, pp. 320-324.

Cathelineau, X., Cahill, D., Widmer, H., Rozet, F., Baumert, H. & Vallancien, G. (2004). Transperitoneal or extraperitoneal approach for laparoscopic radical prostatectomy: a false debate over a real challenge. *J Urol*. 171, 2004, pp. 714-716.

Curto, F., Benijts, J., Pansadoro, A., Barmoshe, S., Hoepffner, J.L. & Mugnier C. (2006). Nerve sparing laparoscopic radical prostatectomy: our technique. *Eur Urol*. 49, 2006, pp. 344-352.

De La Rosette, J.J., Abbou, C.C., Rassweiler, J., Laguna, M.P. & Schulman, C.C. (2002). Laparoscopic radical prostatectomy: a European virus with global potentials. *Arch Esp Urol*. 55, 2002, pp. 603-609.

Gill, I.S. & Zippe, C.D. (2001). Laparoscopic radical prostatectomy: technique. *Urol Clin North Am*. 28, 2001, pp. 423-436.

Guillonneau, B., Cathelineau, X., Barret, E., Rozet, F. & Vallancien, G. (1999). Laparoscopic radical prostatectomy: technical and early oncological assessment of 40 operations. *Eur Urol*. 36, 1999, pp. 14-20.

Guillonneau, B. & Rozet, F. (2002). Perioperative complications of laparoscopic radical prostatectomy: the Montsouris 3-year experience. *J Urol*. 167, 1, 2002 Jan, pp. 51–56.

Guillonneau, B., Cathelineau, X., Doublet, J.D., Baumert, H. & Vallancien, G. (2003). Laparoscopic radical prostatectomy: assessment after 550 procedures. *Crit Rev Oncol Hematol*. 43, 2002, pp. 123-133.

Hoznek, A., Menard, Y., Salomon, L. & Abbou, C.C. Update on laparoscopic and robotic radical prostatectomy. *Curr Opin Urol*. 15, 2005, pp. 173-180.

Humphreys, M.R., Gettman, M.T., Chow, G.K., Zincke, H. & Blute, M.L. (2004). Minimally Invasive Radical Prostatectomy. *Mayo Clin Proc*., 79, 9, Sept 2004, pp. 1169-1180.

Landman, J., Venkatesh, R., Vanlangendonck, R. & Andriole, G.L. (2004). Application of a fixed retraction system to facilitate laparoscopic radical prostatectomy. *J Urol*. 171, 2004, pp. 783-785.

Lein, M., Stibane, I., Mansour, R., Hege, C., Roigas, J. & Wille, A. (2006). Complications, urinary continence, and oncologic outcome of 1000 laparoscopic transperitoneal radical prostatectomies-experience at the Charité Hospital Berlin, Campus Mitte. *Eur Urol*. 50, 2006, pp. 1278-1282; discussion 1283-4.

Levinson, A.W. & Su, L.M. (2007). Laparoscopic radical prostatectomy: current techniques. *Curr Opin Urol,* 17, 2, (Mar 2007), pp.98–103.

Pavlovich, C.P., Trock, B.J., Sulman, A., Wagner, A.A., Mettee, L.Z. & Su, L.M. (2008). 3-year actuarial biochemical recurrence-free survival following laparoscopic radical prostatectomy: experience from a tertiary referral center in the United States. *J Urol.* 179, 2008, pp. 917-921; discussion 921-2.

Raboy, A., Ferzli, G. & Albert, P. (1997). Initial experience with extraperitoneal endoscopic radical retropubic prostatectomy. *Urology.* 50, 1997, pp.849-853.

Rassweiler, J., Sentker, L., Seemann, O., Hatzinger, M., Stock, C. & Frede, T. (2001). Heilbronn laparoscopic radical prostatectomy. Technique and results after 100 cases. *Eur Urol.* 40, 2001, pp.54-64.

Rassweiler, J., Seemann, O., Hatzinger, M., Schulze, M. & Frede, T. (2003). Technical evolution of laparoscopic radical prostatectomy after 450 cases. *J Endourol.* 17, 2003, pp. 143-54.

Rassweiler, J., Hruza, M., Teber, D. & Su, L.M. (2006). Laparoscopic and robotic assisted radical prostatectomy—critical analysis of the results. *Eur Urol.* 49, 2006, pp. 612-624.

Rocco, F., Carmignani, L., Acquati, P., Gadda, F., Dell'Orto, P. & Rocco, B. (2007). Early continence recovery after open radical prostatectomy with restoration of the posterior aspect of the rhabdosphincter. *Eur Urol.* 52, 2007, pp. 376-383.

Rosenblatt, A., Bollens, R. & Espinoza Cohen, B. (2008). Extraperitoneal laparoscopic radical prostatectomy, In: *Manual of Laparoscopic Urology,* Springer-Verlag, ISBN 978-3-540-74726-0 , Berlin Heidelberg, pp. 63-89.

Schuessler, W.W., Kavoussi, L.R., Clayman, R.V. & Vancaille, T. (1992). Laparoscopic radical prostatectomy: initial case report. *J Urol.* 147, 1992, pp. 147: 246A, Abstract no. 130.

Schuessler, W.W., Schulam, P.G., Clayman, R.V. & Kavoussi, L.R. (1997). Laparoscopic radical prostatectomy: initial short-term experience. *Urology.* 50, 1997, pp. 854-857.

Steinberg, A.P. & Gill, I.S. (2004). Laparoscopic prostatectomy: A promising option in the treatment of prostate cancer.*Cleveland Clinic Journal of Medicine.* 71, 2, 2004, pp. 113-121.

Stolzenburg, J.U., Rabenalt, R., Ho, K., Dorschner, W. & Waldkirch, E. (2005). Endoscopic extraperitoneal radical prostatectomy: oncological and functional results after 700 procedures. *J Urol.* 174, 2005, pp. 1271-5; discussion 1275.

Türk, I., Deger, S., Winkelmann, B., Schönberger, B. & Loening, S.A. (2001). Laparoscopic radical prostatectomy. Technical aspects and experience with 125 cases. *Eur Urol.* 40, 2001, pp. 46-52; discussion 53.

Vallancien, G. & Guillonneau, B. (2002). *Laparoscopic Radical Prostatectomy,* Ecole Européenne de Chirurgie Collection, ISBN 2-913487-10-6, Paris, France.

Walsh, P.C. (2000). Radical prostatectomy for localized prostate cancer provides durable cancer control with excellent quality of life: a structured debate. *J Urol.* 163, 2000, pp. 1802-1807.

3

Robot-Assisted Radical Prostatectomy

Jorn H Witt, Vahudin Zugor, Christian Wagner,
Andreas Schutte and Apostolos P Labanaris
*Department of Urology and Pediatric Urology,
Prostate Center Northwest, St. Antonius-Hospital, Gronau,
Germany*

1. Introduction

Over the last decade, robot-assisted radical prostatectomy (RARP) has become a common used surgical procedure for the treatment of prostate cancer (PCa) (35,41). Nowadays, it is considered the dominant approach to radical prostatectomy (RP) in the United States, in European countries such as Belgium and Sweden as well as in other regions where health economic conditions permit (2,12,29).

2. Anatomical considerations

The aim of radical prostatectomy is not only to achieve optimal oncological outcomes but also to preserve the functional aspects of continence and potency (23). In order to achieve this goal, a profound understanding of the prostate anatomy as well as the pelvic anatomy of the surrounding structures is mandatory. Especially, regarding the functional aspects of continence and potency, the ongoing understanding of the anatomical structures and functional principles will surely lead to new unknown aspects in the future. Walz et al have described the contemporary anatomy of the prostate and its surrounding structures in detail in 2010 (37).

3. Patient selection

Patient selection is the same as for the open or standard laparoscopic variants of RP and has been previously described in evidence-based guidelines. Patients exhibiting a clinically localized disease, an expected negative surgical margin status and an individual life expectancy of more than 10 years are three principle indications to perform RP (10,39).

4. Patient preparation

Bowel preparation is used in most institutions and can be achieved with a mild laxative or rectal preparation by enema (34). The surgical field is shaved from the pubic bone to the xiphoid. We prefer preparation of the umbilicus with an alcoholic swab two hours before the procedure and a single shot perioperative antibiotic prophylaxis.

5. Port placement

The port placement is shown in figure 1. Either Verres needle or camera port placement under direct vision in "Hasson technique" is a possible. We prefer the Hasson technique with minilaparatomy and camera port placement above or on the left side of the umbilicus under vision. After establishment of the pneumoperitoneum the robotic and assistant ports are placed under direct vision. After prior abdominal surgery a standard laparoscopic or robotic assisted adhesiolysis could be necessary. Alternatively to the transperitoneal approach, which is being preferred in our institution, an extraperitoneal approach is possible and may be considered in patients with history of e.g. peritonitis (17). The ports are then usually placed about 2cm lower than in the transperitoneal approach. After port placement the patient is placed in a 30 - 40 degrees Trendelenburg position (in case of extraperitoneal approach 20 degrees Trendelenburg is adequate) (28). The patient side cart of the robot is docked and the instruments are inserted under direct vision.

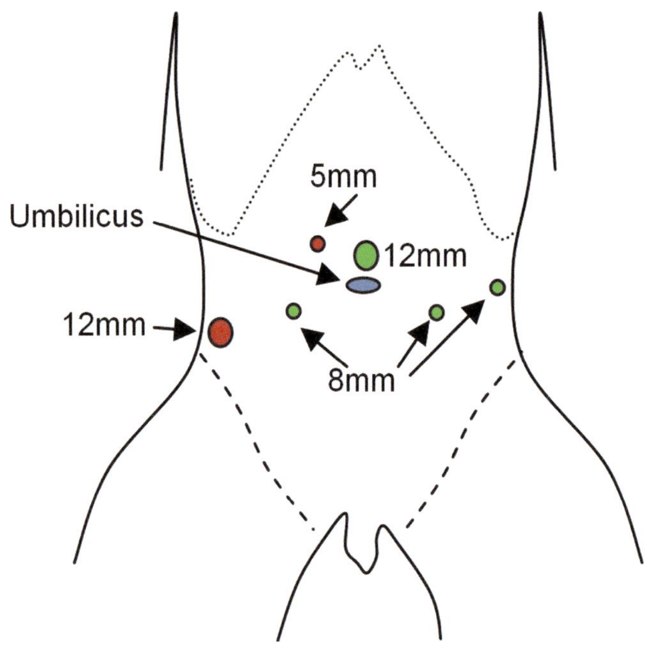

Fig. 1. Port placement

6. Preparation of cavum recii and ventral aspect of the prostate

The preparation begins in the midline, close to the umbilicus, by incising the peritoneum and releasing the bladder from the ventral abdominal wall. On both sides the ligamenta umbilicale mediale are disected after coagulation. The lateral limit of the preparation is the vas deferens at the crossing above the iliac artery. We use a monopolar scissor on the right hand as well as a P.K. dissector for preparation and bipolar coagulation on the left hand. On the third arm we use for retraction purposes a Prograsp. The procedure could also be performed with the use of only two robotic instrument arms, but leads to the need for a second assistant to apply the appropriate traction needed to the structures. In our opinion the use of all three robotic instrument arms is very useful. The preparation is then continued to the pubic bone and the symphysis. The periprostatic fat is removed and separately send to the pathologist revealing in some cases lymph nodes.

7. Incision of the endopelvic fascia

The endopelvic fascia is prepared on both sides and incised, beginning at the base (figure 2). The pelvic floor muscles are separated on both sides from the prostate. In selected cases, the endopelvic fascia on the side where PCa was not detected through the biopsy, can be left intact. The incision of the endopelvic fascia allows better vision of the contour of the prostate and is in our hands preferred in most cases. The preparation is performed apically to the pubovesicle ligaments which are incised close to the prostate.

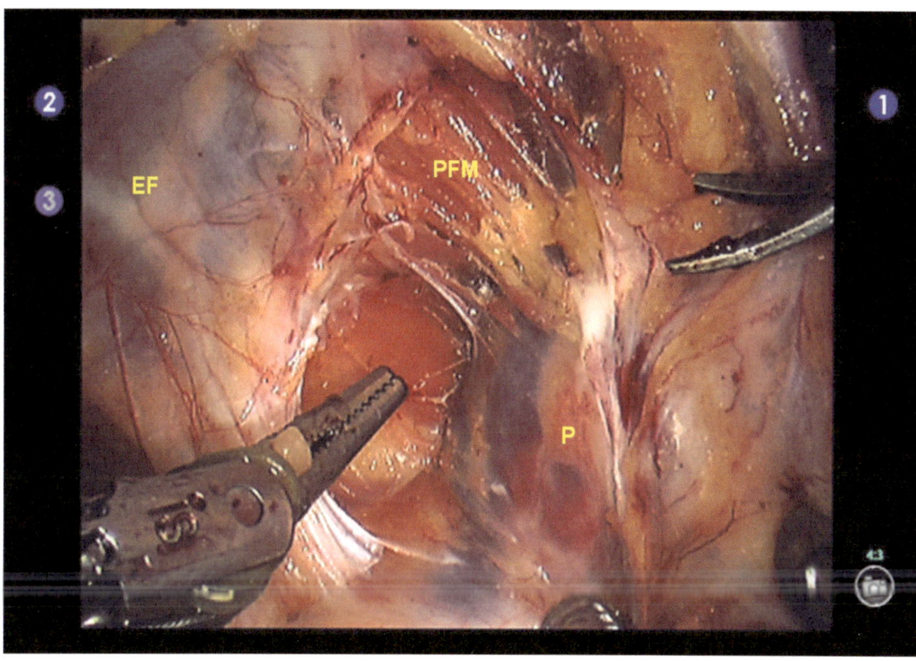

Fig. 2. Incision of the endopelvic fascia on the left side (EF = endopelvic fascia, PFM = pelvic floor muscle, P = Prostate)

8. Dorsal vascular complex

The dorsal vascular complex (DVC) is exposed and ligated with a 2/0 monofilic polyglyconate suture on a CT1 needle. Also stapling techniques or a none suturing techniques have been described (32). For better exposure of the apex during the further preparation and for less bleeding we prefer the suturing of the DVC.

9. Suspension stitch

With the same needle and suture we perform a suspension stitch of the DVC and the pubovesicle ligaments at the periost of the symphysis. Some authors found that this maneuver leads to a better result in early continence. Although the level of evidence for this manoeuvre is not high, it could also be considered as a back up stitch for the DVC. Then a third stitch is additionally performed close to the bladder neck on the dorsal aspect of the prostate. This suture allows better visualization of the bladder neck for the preparation that follows.

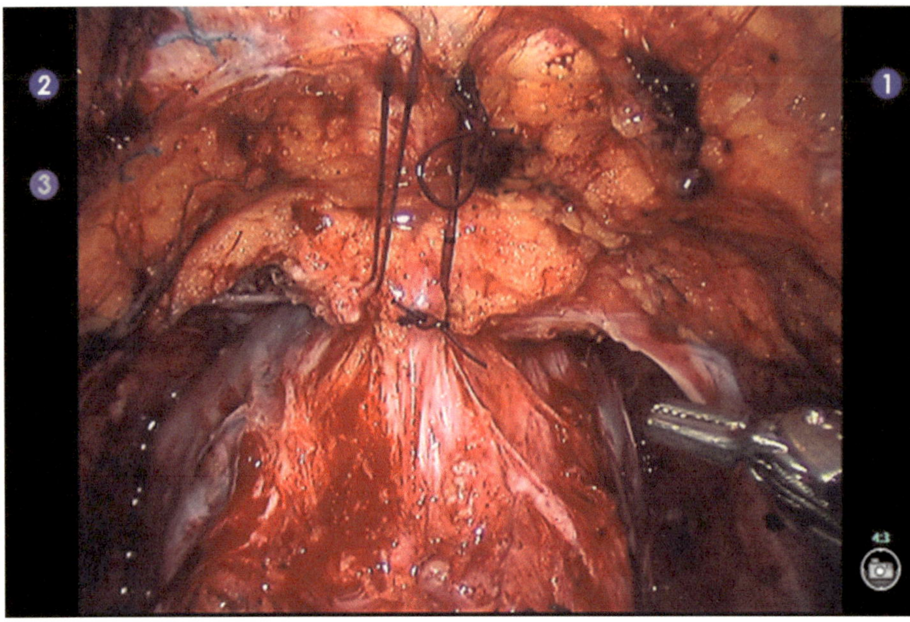

Fig. 3. Suspension stitch

10. Bladder neck preparation

The preparation in now continued between the prostate and bladder. The bladder neck is exposed be indentifying its longitudinal muscular fibers. Lateral to the bladder neck, veins of the DVC can be indentified and coagulated or clipped. We usually use 5 or 10 mm Hemolock clips. In most cases, arteries are also present lateral to the bladder neck, which can be as well coagulated or clipped. The Prograsp is in this step of the procedure a very useful device by keeping traction on the bladder in the cranial direction. In most cases a bladder neck sparing procedure is possible (14). After preparation of the bladder neck, the bladder neck is dorsally incised and the catheter elevated ventrally above the symphysis. Then the dorsal aspect of the bladder neck is incised and the bladder released from the prostate. Incision of the prostate with median lobe should be excluded by identifying the "drop off" phenomenon (Figure 5). The view inside the bladder should be in the dorsal direction. If this is not the case a median lobe should be considered. In case of a bladder neck sparing procedure the orifices usually don't have to be identified. After previous TURP or in patients with a large median lobe, a bladder neck sparing procedure is not possible. Similar situations may be encountered in locally advanced cancers into the bladder. Excision of the bladder up to the orifices in order to achieve a negative surgical margin status is possible. In such cases a consecutively stenting of the ureters and bladder neck reconstruction may be necessary.

11. Preparation of the vas deferens and the seminal vesicles

After releasing the bladder from the prostate the vesicoprostatic muscle is identified. This structure has longitudinal fibers between the region of the trigonum and the prostate ventrally of the level of the vas deferens. Due to the fact that the neurovascular structures, which are important for the erectile function, may be close to the seminal vesicles, this muscle should be incised cold.

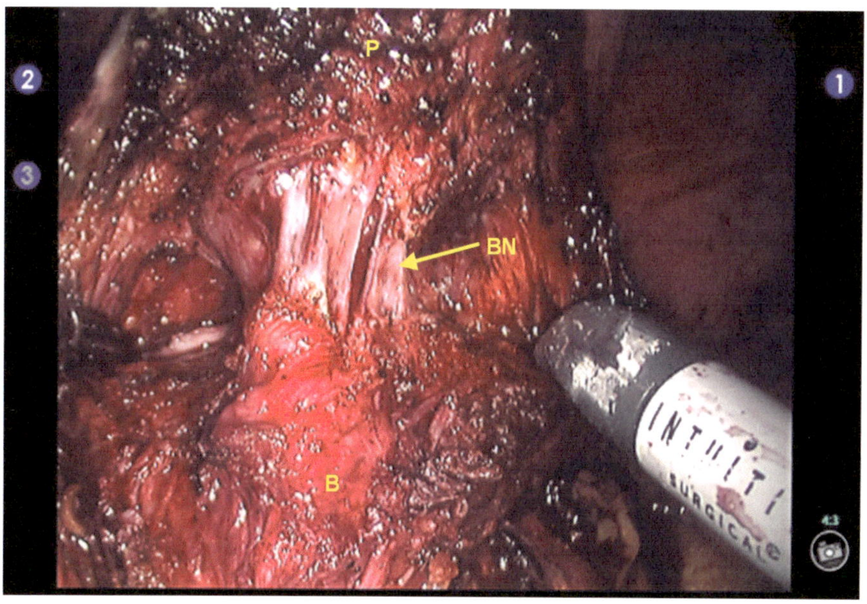

Fig. 4. Bladder neck preparation (B = bladder, BN = bladder neck, P = prostate)

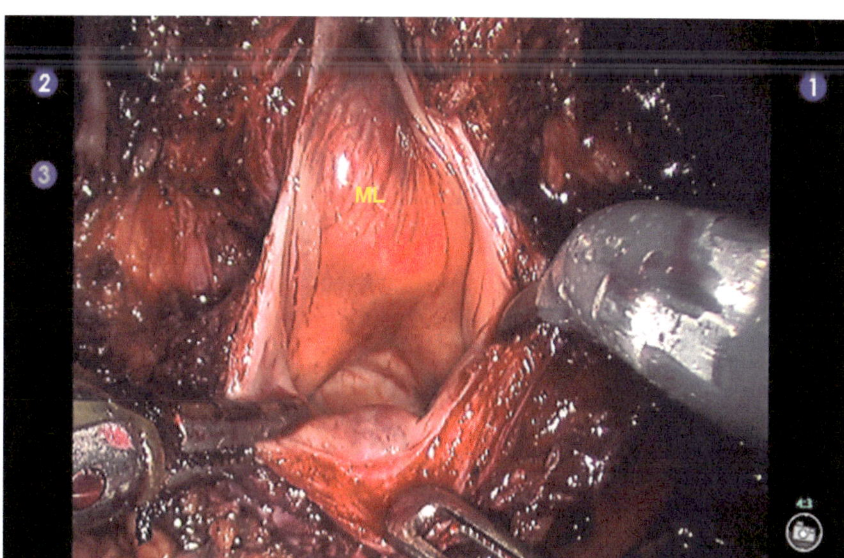

Fig. 5. Drop off (ML = median lobe)

Likewise, all further steps of the procedure are performed without the use of thermal energy to avoid damage of the neurovascular structures, especially in patients with a good erectile function. After the incision of the vesicle prostatic muscle the vas deferens can be identified and lifted up with the Prograsp. With this maneuver the preparation of the seminal vesicles is simplified (Figure 6). From the medial side of the vas deferens the seminal vesicle fascia can be incised and the preparation can be performed to the tips of the seminal vesicles. The vas deferens is then clipped and the seminal vesicle is lifted up in a ventral direction for further preparation. The vessels in the region of the tips of the seminal vesicles are clipped and divided. Preparation is performed on both sides laterally and until the base of the prostate is reached. Usually, laterally to the seminal vesicles, an additional small artery can be identified and should be clipped. Some authors have described the technique of leaving the tips of the seminal vesicles inside to protect the neurovascular structures at the tips of the seminal vesicle.

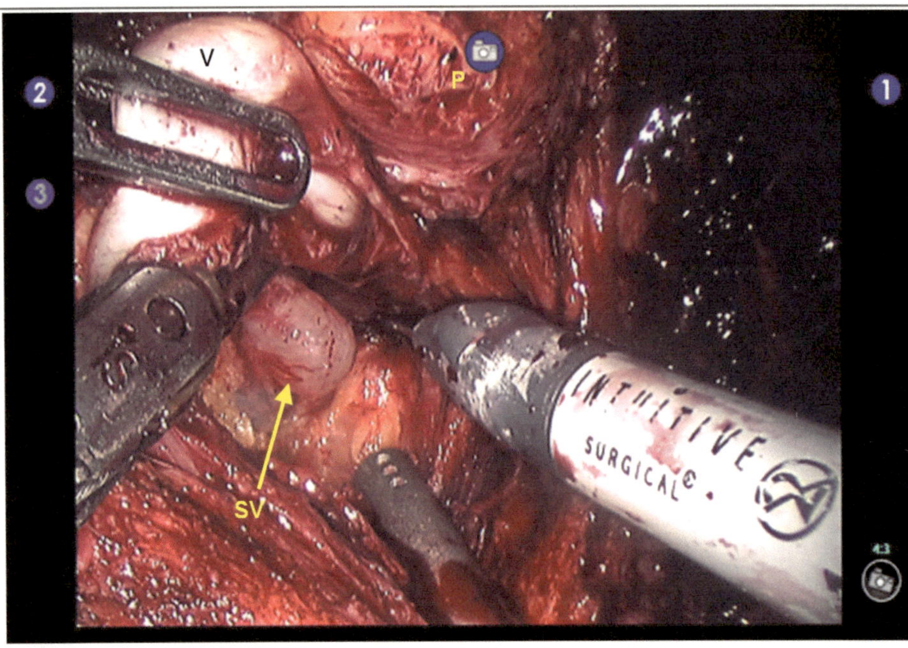

Fig. 6. Seminal vesical preparation on the left side (P = prostate, SV = seminal vesicle, V = Vas)

12. Dorsal preparation of the prostate

At this point the left seminal vesicle is pulled in cranioventrally direction with the Prograsp instrument, the same manoeuvre is performed with a French grasper by the assistant on the right side. The dorsal prostatic fascia, also known as the Denonvilliers fascia, is identified and incised. The dorsal prostatic fascia is in most situations a multilayer fascia and especially in low risk cancer situations can be left on the rectum. This technique gives an additional dorsally support which may help to achieve a good early continence situation. Preparation is performed until the apex of the prostate is reached.

13. Pedicles and neurovascular structures (bundle)

At this point the right base of the prostate is lifted with the Prograsp in left lateral direction and the right pedicle is exposed. In cases where a nerve sparing procedure is possible the lateral prostatic fascia is incised ventrally on the prostate and the preparation of the pedicle is performed close to the base of the prostate. The prostatic blood supply is identified and clipped. Afterwards the neurovascular structures are separated from the prostate by leaving the capsule of the prostate intact. These neurovascular structures are located on the lateral aspect of the prostate, often starting high ventrally and covering the prostate to the dorsal side. In most cases these important structures have the shape of a veil or sheath covering the whole lateral aspect of the prostate. In our opinion the term bundle should be avoided. In low risk patients the preparation can be performed close to the prostate in an intrafascial approach (Figure 7), in medium risk patients the preparation can be performed in an interfascial way by leaving the small artery which travels laterodorsally on the prostate on the specimen. If an extraprostatic extension is visible or in high risk patients a wide resection of the neurovascular structures should be performed. Likewise, the same steps are performed on the left side. Here the Prograsp is used as a hook to retract the bladder. The tableside assistant uses the French grasper to lift the prostate in cranial and lateral direction. Alternatively the release of the neurovascular structures can be performed in a retrograde way, similar to the retropubic radical prostatectomy.

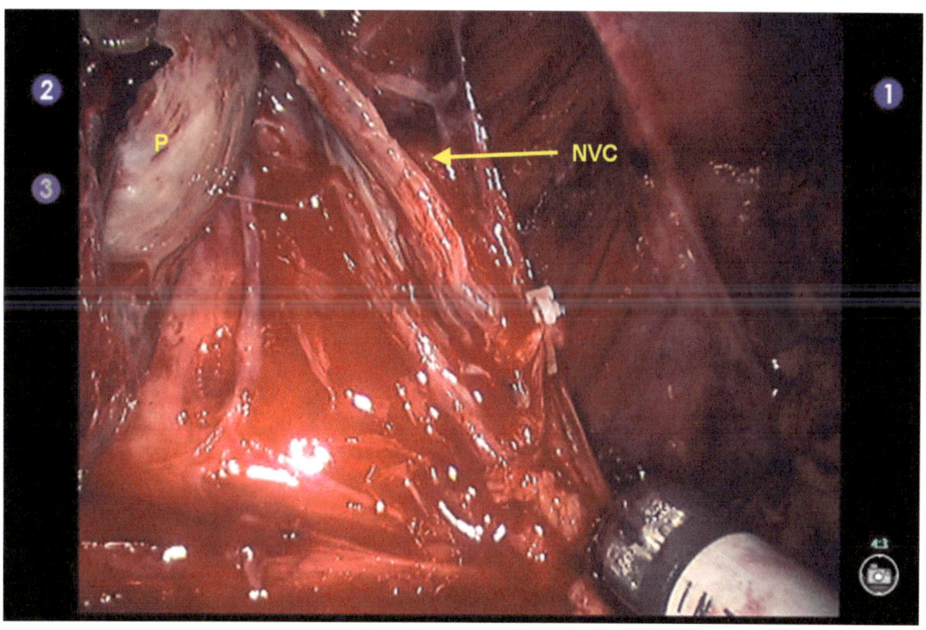

Fig. 7. Released neurovascular complex (NVC = neurovascular complex, P = prostate)

14. Apical dissection

At this point the prostate remains only fixed on the urethra and the dorsal vascular complex. Traction is supplied on the prostate in a cranially direction and the dorsal vascular complex is divided. It is of crucial importance to respect the shape of the prostate to preserve as much as possible functional tissue of the urethra and the surrounding structures for good early continence and also late continence results (31). The urethra is exposed ventrally (Figure 8) and laterally on both sides and then incised on the ventrally half of the circumference. The catheter is removed and the dorsal part of the urethra divided. Remaining adhesions at the level of the dorsal prostatic fascia are finally divided. The specimen is then placed in a retrieval bag. In cases of lymph node dissection, the removal of the nodes can be performed prior to the anastomosis, thus allowing the placement of all dissected specimens in one retrieval bag.

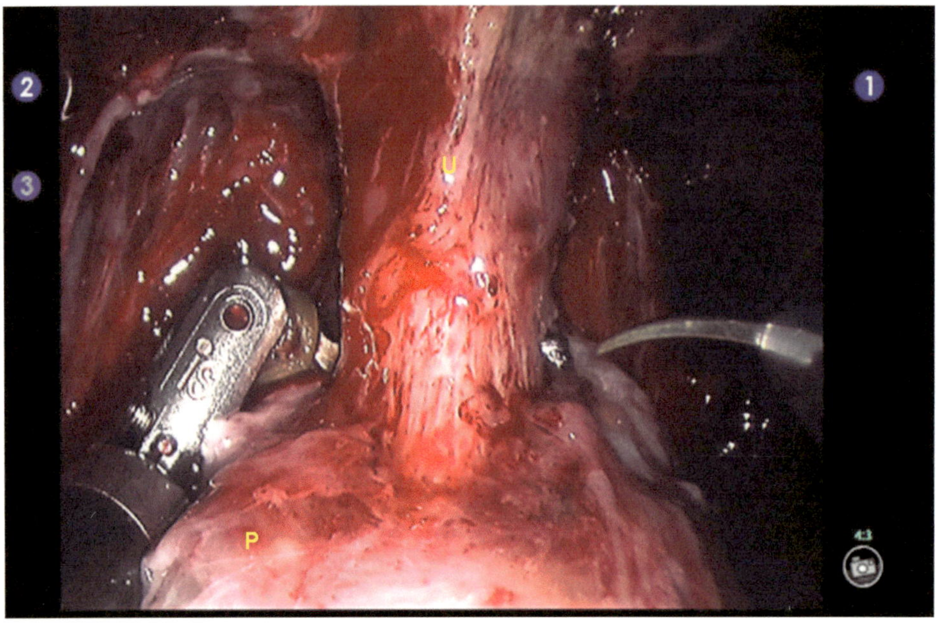

Fig. 8. Apical preparation (P = prostate, U = urethra)

15. Anastomosis

The anastomosis can be performed in a single knot technique or as preferred in our hands and most other institutions in a running suture technique. We use a 19cm double armed barbed suture (polyglyconate 4-0 on an RB1 needle). The first two stitches of the anastomosis are performed at 5 o'clock on the bladder, followed by a stitch at the urethra at 5 o'clock in an inside-out fashion followed by a 6 o'clock stitch outside-in on the bladder, followed by a stitch on the same position at the urethra. After performing a third stitch on the bladder side at 7 o'clock the bladder is approximated to the urethra. In order to achieve a better dorsal stabilization, the dorsal prostatic fascia at the urethral side as well as at the level of the seminal vesicles, is also included during anastomosis (dorsal reconstruction).

A dorsal reconstruction can be also performed solitary. Nevertheless, when comparing both techniques we did not find any differences in postoperative continence results as well as strictures or leakage at day 3-5. The anastomosis is then continued on the left side up to approximately 11 o'clock. The barbed wire can be pulled only in one direction so the approximation of the structures is easier to perform. Alternatively the use of a monofilic polyglyconate suture (3-0) is also possible. Afterwards the right side part of the anastomosis is performed in a similar fashion. The two parts of the suture are then knotted together to complete the anastomosis. At the end of the procedure checking of all possible bleeding sites after reducing the intraabdominal pressure should be performed. We also check the anastomosis by filling the bladder with 200cc of saline. If there is any doubt that the anastomosis might be insufficient, a drain should be placed, in all other cases this is not necessary.

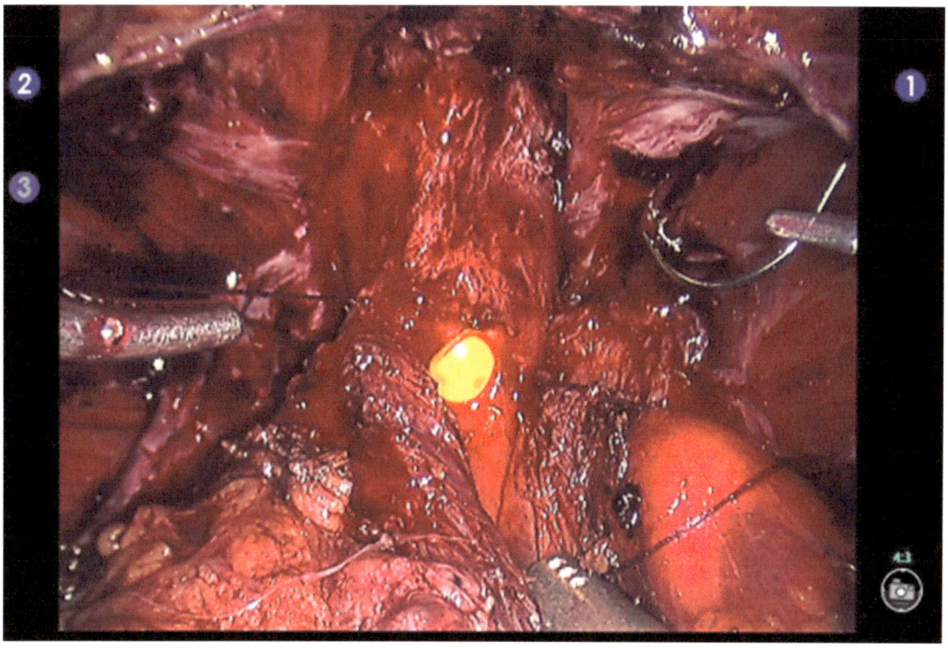

Fig. 9. Anastomosis: left side complete, beginning of the right side.

16. Special considerations

16.1 Bladder neck reconstruction

In cases where a bladder neck sparing procedure is not possible and the bladder neck is wide, a bladder neck reconstruction is necessary. This is often the case after TURP and may also be evident in a large median lobe or in advanced cancer situations with the need of a partial bladder excision. Although several techniques of bladder neck reconstruction have been described, it can be performed in a tennis-racket fashion like as in open surgery, ventrally at the end of the anastomosis or, as we prefer, lateral on both sides. Alternatively also a ventral bladder neck reconstruction is possible. In our opinion the most important goal of the bladder neck reconstruction is not the adjustment of the diameter of the bladder neck to the urethra but the lateralization of the orifices from the anastomosis. For this reason we prefer a both side lateral bladder neck reconstruction beginning on each lateral aspects of the bladder neck in a continuous fashion with 3-0 polyglyconate monofilic suture. In this running suture technique the orifices will be lateralized from the side of the anastomosis.

16.2 Stenting of the ureters

In situations where it is necessary to resect the bladder near to the orifices a stenting of the ureters should be considered. This could be done easily by placing a hydrophilic stiff guide wire into the ureter up to the pyelon and stenting the ureter afterwards with the double J-stent. The aforementioned described bladder neck reconstruction should be performed afterwards. The stent could be left in place for 2 - 4 weeks or could also be removed after the bladder neck reconstruction has been performed.

17. Lymph node dissection

In situations where lymph node dissection is necessary, the nodes can be removed at the beginning of the procedure, before performing the anastomosis or at the end of the procedure. We usually perform the lymph node dissection after the removing of the prostate, this allows us to use a possible waiting time for frozen sections to perform the lymph node dissection. The lymph nodes on the external iliac artery, the extern iliac vein and the fossa obturatoria are removed. The lymphatic vessels should be clipped. In T3 cancers also an extended lymph node dissection up to the aortic bifurcation could be easily performed in a transperitoneal approach (42). Care should be taken of the obturator nerve, the ureters and additional obturatic vessels which can be found in many cases.

18. Postoperative care

At the end of the procedure we change the transurethral catheter, in selected cases also a suprapubic tube could be inserted and the transurethral catheter can be removed on the first postoperative day. The patient should be mobilized on the day of surgery, on the first postoperative day the time of mobilization should reach 6 hours. All drains and i.v. tubes are removed on day one in most of the patients. Only the transurethral catheter is left in place. By suturing the skin and with an additional gluing of the skin the patient can take a shower on the first postoperative day. The patient can be discharged from the medical point of view on postoperative day 1 (38). We usually discharge the patient on day 6 postoperatively after removing of the catheter on day 5. We also perform routinely a cystogram, but with a extravasation rate of lower than 3% a cystogram can also be reserved for special situations. We administer a laxans on postoperative day 1 and also prescribe pelvic floor exercises. The patient is advised avoiding heavy lifting (more than 10kg) and cycling for 4 weeks.

19. Complications

19.1 Intraoperative complications

A bowel lesion, especially in patients who have a history of prior surgery, may occur and can be repaired by suturing easaly. Rectal injuries, a typical complication observed in retropubic RP, is very rare with an incidence of less than 0.2% in our series. In case of a small bowel or a rectal injury and an intraoperative repair we place a drain, but don't change the postoperative procedure.

Intraoperative lesion of iliac vein or artery can be repaired directly and the repair is robotic-assisted usually no problem.

Clipping of the obturator nerve during lymphadenectomy may happen, especially on the left side, titanium clips can be removed easily, Hemolock clips must be cut with a hook scissor on the opposite end of the lock. If this is done no permanent damage of the nerve will occur.

At the end of the procedure all possible sites of bleeding (pedicles, dorsal vascular complex, and iliac vessels) should be checked before undocking the robot by reducing the intraperitoneal pressure to zero. The trocars should be removed under direct visions to check for bleeding from trocar sites. All trocar sites larger than 8mm should be closed at the level of the fascia. This avoids port-site hernias.

19.2 Postoperative complications

19.2.1 Urinary extravasation

If the cystogram shows an extravasation the catheter is left inside for additional 10 days, the catheter can then be removed with or without an additional cystogram (8). If there is a large urinary extravasation with urine in the peritoneal cavity there is a high risk of peritonitis, in these cases a stenting of the ureters and maybe an additional percutaneous drainage of the ureters may be necessary. If there is any doubt of a urinary peritonitis this should be performed immediately. Depending on the case, and although endoscopic management of this situation is possible, open surgery should also be considered.

19.2.2 Postoperative bleeding

In hemodynamic instable patients a postoperative bleeding should be considered and can be evaluated by ultrasound or CT-scan (8). Laparoscopic, robotic assisted or open revision may be necessary to remove the hematoma and take care of the bleeding.

19.2.3 Postoperative subileus

In about 5% of the patients, bowel movement back to normal conditions is delayed (30). This could be avoided by earlier mobilization of the patient, oral fluid intake of about 2.5 litres per day and administering a laxative. In our series, the need of surgical intervention for this phenomenon was never observed.

19.2.4 Early port hernia

Port-site hernias lead to pain at the site of the hernia and could be diagnosed with a CT-scan (25). Open or laparoscopic repair is necessary. We never encountered early port-site hernias since we close the fascia in all ports larger than 8mm.

19.2.5 Late port hernias

Late port-site hernias may occur especially in the site of the specimen removal, usually a mesh repair is required (24).

19.2.6 Non-recognized bowel injuries

The clinical symptoms of an unrecognized bowel injury are often milder than in open surgery. Pain and tension is often found in the port-site close to the injury (13). Open surgical repair is usually required.

20. Conclusion

Robotic assisted radical prostatectomy is a widely used and standardized procedure with excellent oncological and functional results, especially in experienced hands (9,19). The magnification of 10 to 20 times, the excellent degrees of freedom for movement of the

instruments and the intuitive handling of the machine are advantages compared with the open or standard laparoscopic approaches (7,27,33,36). Although evidence for better oncological and functional results are still unproven robotic assisted radical prostatectomy (1,3,15,21,26,39) is in many countries now the standard of care for the surgical removal of the prostate (4,6,22). Transfusion rates are lower and return to normal activity is shorter in RARP (5,16,20). In addition, complex situations like salvage RP or a history of rectum extirpation are no longer a contraindication for RARP (11,18).
In the future the development of new instruments and the possibility of the use of simultaneous imaging will lead to more possibilities and maybe also to better results.

21. References

[1] Atug F, Castle EP, Woods M, Srivastav SK, Thomas R, Davis R. Transperitoneal versus extraperitoneal robotic-assisted radical prostatectomy: is one better than the other? Urology. 2006 Nov;68(5):1077-81.
[2] Badani KK, Kaul S, Menon M. Evolution of robotic radical prostatectomy: assessment after 2766 procedures. Cancer. 2007 Nov 1;110(9):1951-8.
[3] Barocas DA, Salem S, Kordan Y, Herrell SD, Chang SS, Clark PE, Davis R, Baumgartner R, Phillips S, Cookson MS, Smith JA Jr. Robotic assisted laparoscopic prostatectomy versus radical retropubic prostatectomy for clinically localized prostate cancer: comparison of short-term biochemical recurrence-free survival. J Urol. 2010 Mar;183(3):990-6.
[4] Bolenz C, Gupta A, Hotze T, Ho R, Cadeddu JA, Roehrborn CG, Lotan Y. Cost comparison of robotic, laparoscopic, and open radical prostatectomy for prostate cancer. Eur Urol. 2010 Mar;57(3):453-8.
[5] Carmignani L, Pavesi M, Picozzi S. Comparison of transfusion requirements between open and robotic-assisted laparoscopic radical prostatectomy. BJU Int. 2011 Mar;107(5):853-4
[6] Cathelineau X, Sanchez-Salas R, Barret E, Rozet F, Vallancien G. Is laparoscopy dying for radical prostatectomy? Curr Urol Rep. 2008 Mar;9(2):97-100.
[7] Coelho RF, Chauhan S, Palmer KJ, Rocco B, Patel MB, Patel VR. Robotic-assisted radical prostatectomy: a review of current outcomes. BJU Int. 2009 Nov;104(10):1428-35.
[8] Coelho RF, Palmer KJ, Rocco B, Moniz RR, Chauhan S, Orvieto MA, Coughlin G, Patel VR. Early complication rates in a single-surgeon series of 2500 robotic-assisted radical prostatectomies: report applying a standardized grading system. Eur Urol. 2010 Jun;57(6):945-52.
[9] Correa JJ, Pow-Sang JM. Optimizing cancer control and functional outcomes following robotic prostatectomy. Cancer Control. 2010 Oct;17(4):233-44.
[10] Douaihy YE, Sooriakumaran P, Agarwal M, Srivastava A, Grover S, Mudaliar K, Rajan S, Lawlor A, Leung R, Tewari A. A cohort study investigating patient expectations and satisfaction outcomes in men undergoing robotic assisted radical prostatectomy. Int Urol Nephrol. 2010 Aug 11. [Epub ahead of print]
[11] Eandi JA, Link BA, Nelson RA, Josephson DY, Lau C, Kawachi MH, Wilson TG. Robotic assisted laparoscopic salvage prostatectomy for radiation resistant prostate cancer. J Urol. 2010 Jan;183(1):133-7

[12] Finkelstein J, Eckersberger E, Sadri H, Taneja SS, Lepor H, Djavan B. Open Versus Laparoscopic Versus Robot-Assisted Laparoscopic Prostatectomy: The European and US Experience. Rev Urol. 2010 Winter;12(1):35-43.
[13] Fischer B, Engel N, Fehr JL, John H. Complications of robotic assisted radical prostatectomy. World J Urol. 2008 Dec;26(6):595-602.
[14] Freire MP, Weinberg AC, Lei Y, Soukup JR, Lipsitz SR, Prasad SM, Korkes F, Lin T, Hu JC. Anatomic bladder neck preservation during robotic-assisted laparoscopic radical prostatectomy: description of technique and outcomes. Eur Urol. 2009 Dec;56(6):972-80.
[15] Frota R, Turna B, Barros R, Gill IS. Comparison of radical prostatectomy techniques: open, laparoscopic and robotic assisted. Int Braz J Urol. 2008 May-Jun;34(3):259-68
[16] Gainsburg DM, Wax D, Reich DL, Carlucci JR, Samadi DB. Intraoperative management of robotic-assisted versus open radical prostatectomy. JSLS. 2010 Jan-Mar;14(1):1-5.
[17] Gettman MT, Hoznek A, Salomon L, Katz R, Borkowski T, Antiphon P, Lobontiu A, Abbou CC. Laparoscopic radical prostatectomy: description of the extraperitoneal approach using the da Vinci robotic system. J Urol. 2003 Aug;170(2 Pt 1):416-9.
[18] Ginzburg S, Hu F, Staff I, Tortora J, Champagne A, Salner A, Shichman SJ, Kesler SS, Wagner JR, Laudone VP.Does prior abdominal surgery influence outcomes or complications of robotic-assisted laparoscopic radical prostatectomy? Urology. 2010 Nov;76(5):1125-9. Epub 2010 Aug 13.
[19] Herrell SD, Smith JA Jr. Robotic-assisted laparoscopic prostatectomy: what is the learning curve? Urology. 2005 Nov;66(5 Suppl):105-7.
[20] Kordan Y, Barocas DA, Altamar HO, Clark PE, Chang SS, Davis R, Herrell SD, Baumgartner R, Mishra V, Chan RC, Smith JA Jr, Cookson MS. Comparison of transfusion requirements between open and robotic-assisted laparoscopic radical prostatectomy. BJU Int. 2010 Oct;106(7):1036-40.
[21] Laurila TA, Huang W, Jarrard DF. Robotic-assisted laparoscopic and radical retropubic prostatectomy generate similar positive margin rates in low and intermediate risk patients. Urol Oncol. 2009 Sep-Oct;27(5):529-33.
[22] Lowrance WT, Tarin TV, Shariat SF. Evidence based comparison of robotic and open radical prostatectomy. ScientificWorldJournal. 2010 Nov 16;10:2228-37. Review.
[23] McCullough TC, Barret E, Cathelineau X, Rozet F, Galiano M, Vallancien G. Role of robotics for prostate cancer. Curr Opin Urol. 2009 Jan;19(1):65-8.
[24] Murphy D, Challacombe B, Elhage O, Dasgupta P. Complications in robotic urological surgery. Minerva Urol Nefrol. 2007 Jun;59(2):191-8.
[25] Murphy DG, Kerger M, Crowe H, Peters JS, Costello AJ. Operative details and oncological and functional outcome of robotic-assisted laparoscopic radical prostatectomy: 400 cases with a minimum of 12 months follow-up. Eur Urol. 2009 Jun;55(6):1358-66.
[26] Ou YC, Yang CR, Wang J, Cheng CL, Patel VR. Comparison of robotic-assisted versus retropubic radical prostatectomy performed by a single surgeon. Anticancer Res. 2009 May;29(5):1637-42.
[27] Patel VR, Coelho RF, Chauhan S, Orvieto MA, Palmer KJ, Rocco B, Sivaraman A, Coughlin G. Continence, potency and oncological outcomes after robotic-assisted radical prostatectomy: early trifecta results of a high-volume surgeon. BJU Int. 2010 Sep;106(5):696-702.

[28] Phong SV, Koh LK. Anaesthesia for robotic-assisted radical prostatectomy: considerations for laparoscopy in the Trendelenburg position. Anaesth Intensive Care. 2007 Apr;35(2):281-5.

[29] Scales CD Jr, Jones PJ, Eisenstein EL, Preminger GM, Albala DM. Local cost structures and the economics of robot assisted radical prostatectomy. J Urol. 2005 Dec;174(6):2323-9.

[30] Sharma NL, Shah NC, Neal DE. Robotic-assisted laparoscopic prostatectomy. Br J Cancer. 2009 Nov 3;101(9):1491-6.

[31] Shikanov SA, Eng MK, Bernstein AJ, Katz M, Zagaja GP, Shalhav AL, Zorn KC. Urinary and sexual quality of life 1 year following robotic assisted laparoscopic radical prostatectomy. J Urol. 2008 Aug;180(2):663-7.

[32] Singh I, Hemal AK. Robotic-assisted radical prostatectomy in 2010. Expert Rev Anticancer Ther. 2010 May;10(5):671-82.

[33] Srivastava A, Grover S, Sooriakumaran P, Joneja J, Tewari AK. Robotic-assisted laparoscopic prostatectomy: a critical analysis of its impact on urinary continence. Curr Opin Urol. 2011 May;21(3):185-94.

[34] Starnes DN, Sims TW. Care of the patient undergoing robotic-assisted prostatectomy. Urol Nurs. 2006 Apr;26(2):129-36.

[35] Sterrett SP, Jarrard DF. Robotic assisted laparoscopic radical prostatectomy: evolution and outcomes. Minerva Urol Nefrol. 2008 Mar;60(1):31-9.

[36] Shikanov SA, Zorn KC, Zagaja GP, Shalhav AL. Urology. 2009 Sep;74(3):619-23. Trifecta outcomes after robotic-assisted laparoscopic prostatectomy.

[37] Walz J, Burnett AL, Costello AJ, Eastham JA, Graefen, M, Guilloneau, B, Manon, M, Montorsi, F, Myers RP, Rocco B, Villers A. A critical analysis of the current knowledge of surgical anatomy to optimization of cancer control and preservation of continence and erection in candidates for radical prostatectomy. European Urology 2010, (57) 179-192.

[38] Watts R, Botti M, Beale E, Crowe H, Costello AJ. Patient outcomes in the acute recovery phase following robotic-assisted prostate surgery: a prospective study. Int J Nurs Stud. 2009 Apr;46(4):442-9.

[39] Williams SB, Hu JC. Salvage robotic assisted laparoscopic radical prostatectomy: indications and outcomes. World J Urol. 2010 Nov 21. [Epub ahead of print]

[40] Wilson T, Torrey R. Open versus robotic-assisted radical prostatectomy: which is better? Curr Opin Urol. 2011 May;21(3):200-5.

[41] Wolfram M, Bräutigam R, Engl T, Bentas W, Heitkamp S, Ostwald M, Kramer W, Binder J, Blaheta R, Jonas D, Beecken WD. Robotic-assisted laparoscopic radical prostatectomy: the Frankfurt technique. World J Urol. 2003 Aug;21(3):128-32.

[42] Yee DS, Katz DJ, Godoy G, Nogueira L, Chong KT, Kaag M, Coleman JA. Extended pelvic lymph node dissection in robotic-assisted radical prostatectomy: surgical technique and initial experience.Urology. 2010 May;75(5):1199-204.

4

Laparoscopic Living Kidney Donation

Leonienke F.C. Dols and Jan N.M. IJzermans
Erasmus MC Rotterdam
The Netherlands

1. Introduction

Kidney transplantation is the therapy of choice for patients with end-stage renal disease and gives the best chance on long-term survival with a good quality of life. Allografts can be procured from living and deceased donors. Since the successful kidney transplantations in the early 1950s by Rene Kuss and Joseph Murray great progress has been made in this field of medicine.[1] With the introduction of adequate immunosuppressive therapy in the 1960s and new organ preservation techniques the outcome of the transplantation procedures using deceased donor kidneys improved significantly and the use of living donors became an exception as the risk of living kidney donor were thought to be unacceptable. Furthermore, in those years there was an adequate number of deceased donors to accommodate the number of patients on the waiting lists.

In the late 80s a growing discrepancy was noted between organ demand and supply due to an increasing number of patients with end-stage renal disease (ESRD) included for transplantation and a stagnating number of organ donors. The average waiting time for a kidney transplant from a deceased donor increased significantly and up to twenty percent of patients on dialysis had to be removed from the waiting list annually because of a worsening condition or even mortality. This encouraged a new interest in live donor kidney transplantation and in the last decade the number of transplants from live donors significantly increased in the Western World. In addition, the use of live kidney donor transplantation created new opportunities, including crossover programs and pre-emptive and ABO-incompatible kidney transplantations. All these developments contributed to the success of live kidney donation at present and popularity is still increasing in many countries. Today the expansion of live kidney donation may be considered as the most realistic option to solve the problem of kidney donor shortage. The ongoing stream of technical innovations and social, ethical and psychological research focused on live kidney donation legitimize the increasing use of living donors.

Renal transplantation from living donors confers several advantages as compared to dialysis and transplantation from deceased donors, including improved longer-term patient survival, better quality of life, immediate functioning of the transplant, better transplant survival, and the possibility of transplanting pre-emptively. To date the health of live kidney donors at long-term follow-up is good, and the procedure is considered to be safe. Due to good outcome of living kidney donors, the boundaries for acceptance of kidney donors are shifting towards a wider acceptance. Donors with higher body mass index (BMI), moderate hypertension, older age or kidneys with multiple arteries are nowadays accepted.[2-8]

Currently, attention to donor wellbeing has become a priority, and therefore the surgical technique must be optimized continually. Surgical practice has evolved from the open lumbotomy, through mini-incision muscle-splitting open (MIDN), to minimally invasive laparoscopic techniques. Over the last years many changes have been introduced in the field of living kidney donor nephrectomy. Laparoscopic donor nephrectomy is now the gold standard. There are different minimally invasive techniques, including standard laparoscopic, hand-assisted laparoscopic, hand-assisted retroperitoneoscopic, pure retroperitoneoscopic, and robotic-assisted live donor nephrectomy. Different centres have different visions and experience on which technique to use. In the literature, there is level I evidence that minimally invasive techniques are preferred above open donor nephrectomy.[9] Optimizing the donation procedure is mainly focused on donor safety and includes proper definition of criteria for inclusion of donors, anaesthetic and surgical aspects and post-operative care. Long-term follow-up may be offered as surveillance program to detect potential threats for the donors health such as hypertension, protein loss or overweight.
In this chapter we'll address the surgical procedure of live kidney donation and discuss aspects that may influence successful outcome.

2. Pre-operative

2.1 Standard evaluation of the donor

Selection of live kidney donors is mixed by ethical and medical issues. It is only justified if the harm to the donor is limited and the potential benefit to the recipient is major. The risk for the short-term and long-term adverse health consequences to the donor is therefore essential. The Amsterdam Forum has established guidelines for the (relative) contra-indications to live kidney donation: donors must have sufficient renal function (GFR more than 80 ml/min), no hypertension (less than 140/90 mm Hg), no obesity (BMI less than 35 kg/m^2), negative urine analysis for protein (less than 300mg/24 hours) and erythrocytes, no diabetes, stone disease, malignancy or urinary tract infections, a minor or no cardiovascular or pulmonary risk and smoking cessation and alcohol abstinence is obligatory. To ensure donor safety, every donor should be offered a number of standard tests, including blood and urine screening , chest x-ray, electrocardiogram (ECG), radiographic assessment of the kidneys and vessels via renal ultrasound, computed tomography (CT) with intravenous contrast or magnetic resonance imaging (MRI) with intravenous contrast, psychological evaluation, and age- and family history–appropriate additional cardiac testing.[10]
A multidisciplinary approach including nephrologists, transplant surgeons, urologists, and psychologists is required to optimize the quality of a live kidney donation program in each hospital. Disciplines have to cooperate in the screening of donors and informing relatives without exerting pressure on potential donors. Each step in the multidisciplinary approach should be optimized. Imaging of the donor kidney should be performed without any complications and the surgical procedure should be organised with optimal peri-operative care to minimize pain and discomfort to the donor. Advances in surgical technique have improved the comfort of the donor considerably and the risks of morbidity and mortality have been minimized.

2.2 Choices in the selection of living kidney donors

2.2.1 Side selection

Meticulous preoperative preparation of donor operations has become increasingly important as vascular anatomy may significantly influence safety and surgical outcome.

Traditionally, the donor's renal anatomy was assessed by angiography with good results but with significant consequences for the donor including radiation and a short stay in the hospital. Magnetic Resonance Imaging (MRI) and Computed Tomography (CT) have both been reported feasible alternatives.[11, 12]Angiography was gradually replaced by MRI as this technique does not cause radiation and, in addition, provides information on venous anatomy. Recently, new CT-protocols allow the use of minimal radiation while offering optimal imaging of the renal anatomy and they may be used safely in the work-up of selected donors.
If both kidneys have a normal or comparable anatomy regarding the number of renal vessels there is the issue of choosing the right or left kidney, especially in those cases where a laparoscopic approach is considered. Right-sided donor nephrectomy has been associated with a shorter renal vein and renal vein thrombosis in the recipient. Reluctance towards the right side arose when Mandal et al. described a worse outcome for right kidneys with significantly more renal vein thrombosis. [13] One RCT, one prospective and some retrospective studies concluded that right sided-donor nephrectomy is also justified, and in some studies indicate the superiority of the right side. [14-21] In theory a shorter renal vein may lead to a more difficult anastomosis, but no studies so far confirmed this concept.
Another issue is the use of kidneys with multiple arteries. The rationale was to avoid vascular and ureteral complications by using only kidneys with single arteries. But as there were doubts about the use of the right kidney, many centres favoured left donor nephrectomy even in the presence of multiple arteries. Live donor kidneys with multiple arteries are associated with increased surgical complexity for removal and increased rate of recipient ureteral complications. Multiple arteries may increase operation time and risk for the donor. Accessory lower pole arteries are associated with a higher rate of recipient ureteral complications indicating the importance of arterial imaging.

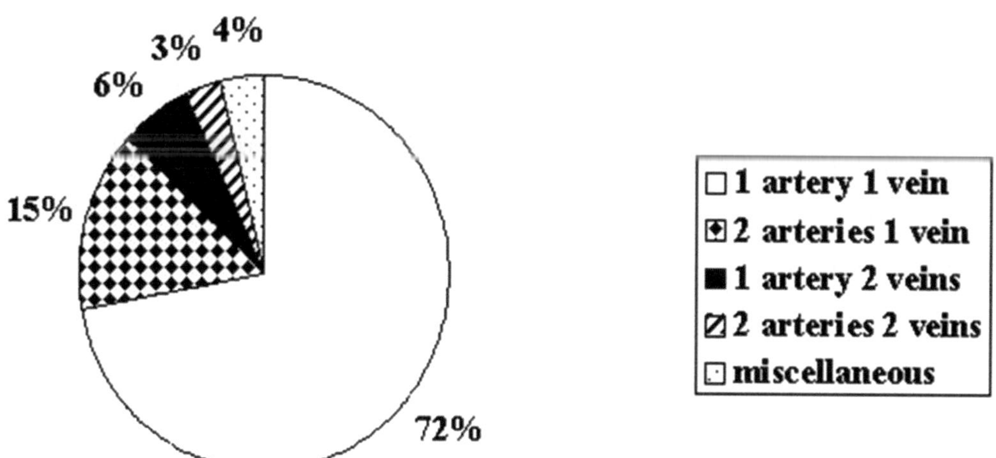

Kok et al, Transplantation. 2008 Jun 27;85(12):1760-5.

Fig. 1. Variation in arterial and venous anatomy

At present there are studies, one prospective and a small number of retrospective studies comparing single and multiple arteries. All studies included a relative small number of donors with multiple arteries and indicate the safety and feasibility of donor nephrectomy in case of multiple arteries. Two studies suggest that multiple renal arteries are associated with more ureteral complications in the recipient, especially when accessory arteries to the lower renal pole are involved. [12, 22-24]

	Single artery (n=138)	Multiple arteries (n=47)	P-value
Warm ischemia time (minutes)	6.0 (2.8)	7.3 (3.1)	0.009
Time until kidney extraction (minutes)	182 (48)	204 (55)	0.023
Skin-to-skin time (minutes)	225 (51)	247 (57)	0.023
Blood loss (ml)	220 (456)	225 (204)	0.029
Intra-operative complications	22 (16%)	7 (15%)	0.864
Postoperative complications	11 (8%)	6 (13%)	0.326
Ureteral complications (recipient)	30 (14%)	14 (21%)	0.127
Ureteral complications leading to re-operation	11 (5%)	7 (11%)	0.096

Kok et al, Transplantation. 2008 Jun 27;85(12):1760-5.

Table 1. Outcomes of procurement of kidneys with single versus multiple arteries by laparoscopic donor nephrectomy. Categorical data are displayed as No. (%) and continuous variables as mean (SD).

2.2.2 Age

Due to the increasing shortage of deceased kidney donors one is trying to expand and maximize the live donor pool. In this transition new criteria are being defined and a number of issues studied as relative contra-indications for the operative procedure include age, body weight and co morbidity of the living donor.
Nowadays, older live donors, obese donors and donors with minor co morbidity indeed may be selected as candidates for kidney donation. There is an ongoing shift towards the acceptance of these donors and the outcome demonstrates the feasibility of this approach in order to bridge the gap between demand and supply of kidney transplants.
Controversy remains, as age related changes in the kidney may result in a decline in renal function over the years, and so far the combination of aging and donor nephrectomy has only been investigated by few. We questioned whether the outcome of older live kidney donation wouldn't hamper the glomerular filtration rate (GFR) on long-term after donation. In addition older donors may also have an increased risk of other perioperative and postoperative complications as they often have a higher 'American Society of Anesthesiologist score' (ASA-score), indicating more comorbidity, a higher incidence of hypertension and a higher Body Mass Index (BMI). All these factors may contribute to a higher risk of complications related to a surgical intervention. Our study demonstrated that the decline in eGFR is similar in younger and older donors. As kidney function does not progressively decline during follow up we believe that, live kidney donation by older donors can be considered safe. Furthermore, we found that graft survival was not compromised in case kidneys from older donors were used.[25-31]

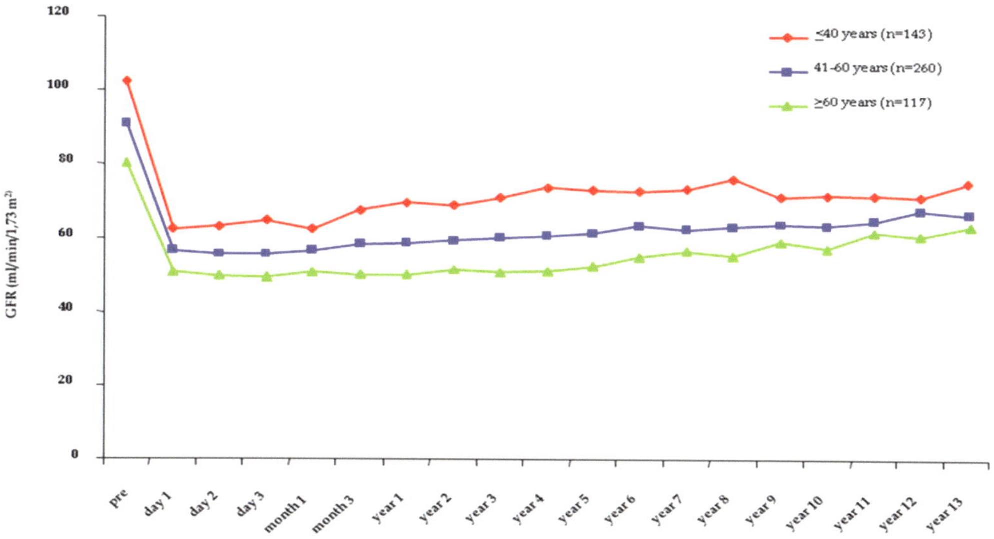

Dols et al. N Engl J Med. 2009 Jan 29;360(5):459-69.

Fig. 2. Glomerular filtrations rate after living donor nephrectomy, divided into age groups.

	Hazard ratio	95%-CI	P-value
BMI donor	1.085	1.029-1.144	0.003
Mismatch-total	1.172	1.025-1.340	0.020
Age donor	1.014	0.995-1.034	0.169
Age recipient	0.988	0.917-1.005	0.210
Gender donor	0.895	0.563-1.423	0.672
Gender recipient	0.906	0.565-1.452	0.810

Dols et al. Am J Transplant. 2011 Apr;11(4):737-42.

Table 2. Multivariate analysis for the association between clinical variables and graft survival.

2.2.3 BMI

To date donors with isolated abnormalities, like obesity, are included in living donation programs. This is a significant challenge for the laparoscopic surgeon. In addition to technical aspects like positioning of the donor, the port-site of the trocars and the instrumentation needed surgeons may face longer and more complex operation procedures with the risk of a higher incidence of anaesthetic and postoperative complications. Studies suggest that laparoscopic donor nephrectomy is safe in selected obese donors. Obese donors have higher baseline cardiovascular risk and warrant risk reduction for long-term health. Furthermore obesity acts on renal function, it accounts for an increase in glomerular filtration rate with less elevated or even decreased effective renal plasma flow, and filtration fraction is increased. The filtration fraction is a predictor for renal function loss, independent of blood pressure. Multiple factors are assumed to contribute to these renal hemodynamic alterations such as insulin resistance, the renin-angiotensin system and the tubulo-glomerular responses to increased proximal sodium reabsorption, and possibly also inappropriate activity of the sympathetic nervous system and increased leptin levels. Together with donor nephrectomy this might be harmful on long-term follow-up, especially because the incidence of overweight and obesity is increasing. While early operative results are encouraging, we advocate careful study of obese donors, especially for the long-term renal effects.

In general, a body mass index (BMI) below 35 is considered acceptable to undergo donor nephrectomy without increased risks. It remains open for discussion which operative procedure should be preferred in obese donors. LDN has been demonstrated feasible in this category of donors and can lead to equivalent results in obese as in normal weight individuals. In specialized centers in the USA, hand-assisted LDN in overweight and obese donors has become a common practice. Nevertheless, total LDN in overweight and obese donors is definitely more challenging and experience is required to render acceptable results. On the other hand, total LDN may avoid postoperative complications that typically occur in obese individuals such as wound infections and incisional hernias, because there is no hand introduced into the abdominal cavity and the extraction incision is smaller as a hand-port is not required. As opposed to many American centers, many European centers are still reluctant towards LDN in general and LDN in donors with more difficult anatomy in particular. [32-36]

	Level of evidence	Type of evidence
Left versus right	II	- RCT - Prospective study - Retrospective studies
Multiple arteries vs single artery	III	- Prospective studies - Retrospective studies
Obese vs non-obese donors	III	-Retrospective study

Dols et al, Transpl Int. 2010 Feb;23(2):121-30.

Table 3. Surgical issues surrounding live kidney donation; level and type of evidence.

3. Intra-operative

3.1 Surgical techniques

Different transplant centers use different techniques. There are a lot of variations in technique, but we tend to describe the most universal way in which these operations are performed. Which surgical technique to use is depending on the preference and experience of the surgeon. In case a surgeon can perform all techniques, minimal invasive techniques are preferred.

3.1.1 Open donor nephrectomy: Flank incision versus mini-incision

With the donor placed in a lateral decubitus position, lumbotomy is performed in the eleventh intercostal space or below the 12th rib. Sometimes a rib resection is mandatory to allow adequate view. The muscles are transected. A mechanical retractor is installed, and the retroperitoneal space opened. The kidney is dissected from its capsula and the arterial and venous structures are identified. After dissection, the ureter is divided and sutured distally. Thereafter, the kidney is extracted, flushed and stored on ice.
Mini-incision muscle-splitting approach (MIDN) is performed with the patient placed in a lateral decubitus position and the operation table maximally flexed. A horizontal 10–15 cm skin incision is made anterior to the 11th rib towards the umbilicus. Sometimes an anterior vertical incision is made in other centres. The fascia and muscles of the abdominal wall are either split attempting to avoid harming the intercostal nerves or divided. The peritoneum is displaced medially. As the working space is limited long instruments have to be used. Further dissection and preparation of the vascular structures is performed as described above.

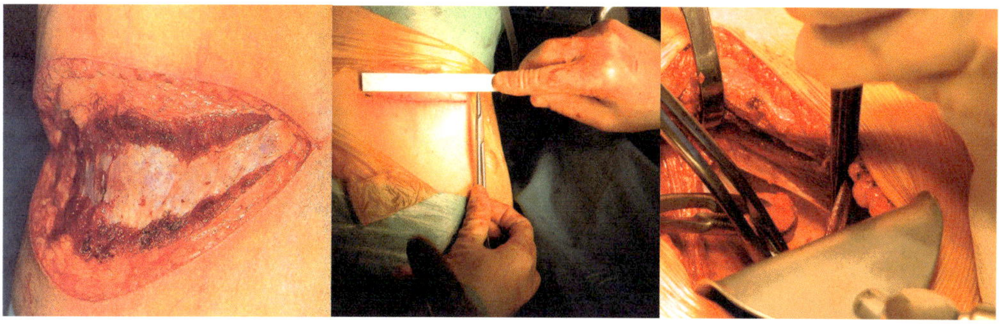

Fig. 3. Flank Incision (left) and mini-incision muscle sparing donor nephrectomy (middle and right).

Conventional open living donor nephrectomy is associated with disincentives including long hospital stay, prolonged postoperative pain, cosmetic problems and long convalescence time. The flank incision technique sometimes required a rib resection, with considerable co-morbidity. There is one randomized controlled trial RCT comparing transcostal to subcostal incision (Level II evidence). Srivastava et al. shows that patients in the subcostal group (n=25) had a lesser postoperative analgesic requirement, shorter hospital stay and shorter convalescence time compared with the ribresection transcostal group (n=24). [37] Mini-incision donor nephrectomy (MIDN) results in similar donor safety, as reflected by the absence of major complications, a similar number of minor intra- and postoperative complications and equivalent graft function. Donors benefit from reduced blood loss, shorter hospitalization, and preservation of continuity of abdominal muscles, only with marginally longer operation time, without compromising graft and recipient survival. Kok et al. described the differences between MIDN and ODN. The median operation time was 158 and 144 min ($p = 0.02$). Blood loss was significantly less after MIDN (median 210 vs. 300 ml, $p = 0.01$). Intra-operatively, 4 (7%) and 1 (1%) bleeding episodes occurred. Postoperatively, complications occurred in 12% in both groups. Hospital stay was 4 and 6 days ($p < 0.001$). In one (2%) and 11 (13%) donors ($p = 0.02$) late complications related to the incision occurred. Neipp at al. found an operating time of 129 min for ODN and 133 min for

MIDN. Blood loss and morphine requirements were not reported. Early complications occurred in 7% following ODN and in 4% following MIDN. Late complications were observed in 21% after ODN and 1% after MIDN. The mean hospital stay was significantly longer following ODN (7.5 vs. 6.4 days). [38, 39]
There is evidence to prefer mini-incision techniques to classic flank incisions (level III). Notwithstanding MIDN was a step forward, there were still disincentives to the open, not minimally invasive approach; this may be a drawback for possible live kidney donors.

3.1.2 Hand-assisted techniques

The hand-assisted laparoscopic (HALDN) and retroperitoneoscopic (HARP) donor nephrectomy start with an incision for the handport. With the HARP technique the retroperitoneal space is created manually (or with a balloon or catheter) through the pfannenstiel incision. An endoscope is introduced and one or two other ports are inserted. The retroperitoneum is insufflated to 12-cm H_2O carbon dioxide pressure. In the HALDN after establishing a pneumoperitoneum, the colon is mobilized and displaced medially. Further dissection and preparation of the vascular structures is performed as described above. The renal artery and vein are divided using an endoscopic stapler and the kidney is removed manually.
Hand-assisted donor nephrectomy can be performed transperitoneally (HALDN) and retroperitoneally (HARP). Hand-assistance can be performed during the whole operation or only during the stapling- and extraction phase, with different incisions for hand introduction. Periumbilical incision, a midline supraumbilical incision, a midline infraumbilical incision, or a Pfannenstiel incision have been described in several studies.
The advantages of hand-assisted donor nephrectomy above conventional laparoscopy include the ability to use tactile feedback, easier and rapid control of bleeding by digital pressure, better exposure and dissection of structures, rapid kidney removal. Overall, these advantages may lead to a shorter skin to skin- and warm ischemia time. With the retroperitoneal approach there is less chance to injure the intra-abdominal organs. This is an important advantage in times where safety of laparoscopic technique is still questioned.
Hand-assisted transperitoneal has been compared to laparoscopic donor nephrectomy. Most studies describing hand-assisted laparoscopic (transperitoneally) donor nephrectomy conclude that the hand-assisted technique is superior to the laparoscopic technique regarding operative time. Blood loss was less, WIT, and hospital stay were shorter for the HALDN. Complications and morphine requirement, convalescence time, and graft and recipient survival were similar in most studies. One randomized controlled trial of Bargmann et al. shows no difference between the two techniques, and an even longer operative time for the hand-assisted laparoscopic technique.[40]
Data on hand-assisted retroperitoneal compared to laparoscopic donor nephrectomy are scarce. Only three studies compare left-sided hand-assisted retroperitoneoscopic with laparoscopic donor nephrectomy. Two centers posed the hand-assisted retroperitoneoscopic approach as an alternative for right-sided donor nephrectomy. Sundqvist et al. performed a prospective study, comparing HARP (n= 11), LDN (n= 14) and open donor nephrectomy (n= 11). Hand-assisted retroperitoneoscopic donor nephrectomy had a significantly shorter operation time compared to LDN (145 min vs 218 minutes, $p<0.05$). Gjertsen et al. performed a retrospective study, comparing HARP (n= 11), LDN (n= 15) and open donor nephrectomy (n= 25). Reduced operation time was observed for the HARP group compared with the LDN (166

min vs 244 min). Wadstrom et al. reported operative time for the HARP (n=18) was significantly shorter than that of the LDN (n=11) (270 vs 141 min). Warm ischemia time was significantly longer in the LDN (297 vs 177 sec). There was no statistically significant difference in operative bleeding or length of hospital stay between the groups. [41-43]

Outcome of most studies comparing different minimal invasive techniques are similar in terms of intra- and post-operative outcome for donor and recipient, and seems promising, but studies are small, too heterogeneous, and with low level of evidence. There is one randomized controlled trial described in literature and done, but not yet published.

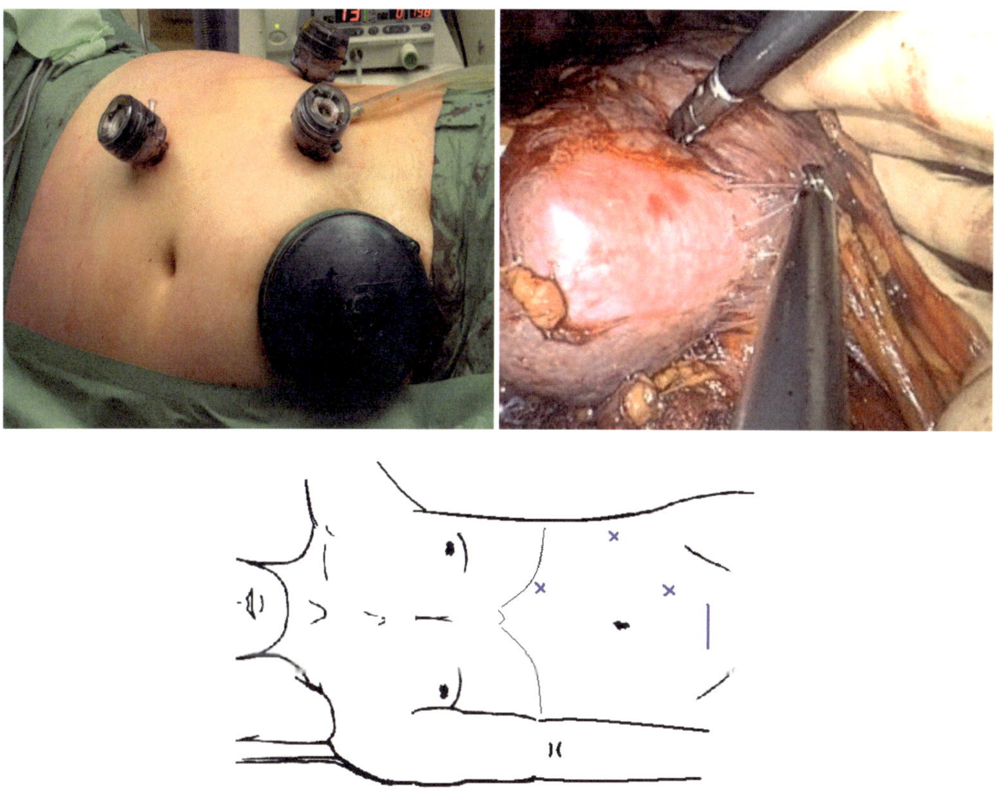

Fig. 4. Hand-assisted retroperitoneal donor nephrectomy and placement of the incisions.

3.1.3 LDN vs ODN

Laparoscopic donor nephrectomy is performed with the donor in lateral decubitus position. In short, a 10-mm trocar is introduced under direct vision. The abdomen is insufflated to 12-cm H_2O carbon dioxide pressure. A 30° video endoscope and 3 to 4 additional trocars are introduced. The colon is mobilized and displaced medially. Opening of the renal capsule and division of the perirenal fat is facilitated using an ultrasonic device or diathermia. After identification and careful dissection of the ureter, the renal artery, and the renal vein, a pfannenstiel incision is made. An endobag is introduced into the abdomen. The ureter is clipped distally and divided. The renal artery and vein are divided using an endoscopic stapler. The kidney is placed in the endobag and extracted through the pfannenstiel incision.

Since MIDN was introduced, evidence has mounted that the laparoscopic approach may be superior to conventional open donor nephrectomy.
Various non-randomized studies have led to the similar conclusion, despite longer operation times and longer warm ischemia time LDN results in shorter hospital stay, faster recovery, less pain, less blood loss, earlier return to work, and better quality of life as compared to the conventional open approach. Most of these studies presented (hand-assisted) laparoscopic donor nephrectomy as an alternative rather than as the preferred technique. Several case series from large volume centres in the United States tried to prove the feasibility and safety of the laparoscopic technique. Leventhal et al. reported a group of 500 patients with an overall rate of intra- and postoperative complications of respectively 2.8% and 3.4%. There were 9 conversions (1.8%), of which 6 were in the first 100 cases. Thirty patients experienced an intraoperative or procedure-related complication (6.0%).[44]
The remaining issues surrounding the use of laparoscopic donor nephrectomy, including long-term follow-up, complications, and donor and recipient safety, are gradually being solved. Nowadays it is the standard technique in a lot of centres for surgeons experienced in laparoscopic techniques. There is level I evidence for the superiority of LDN, but safety remains an issue, and must be adequately studied.

3.1.4 LDN vs MIDN

One RCT, one retrospective study, and one meta-analysis (Level I evidence) aimed to assess the superiority of either the laparoscopic or the minimally invasive open approach (MIDN).
The RCT concluded that laparoscopic donor nephrectomy results in a better quality of life compared with MIDN with equal safety and graft function. Compared to mini incision open donor nephrectomy (n=50), laparoscopic donor nephrectomy (n=50) resulted in longer skin-to-skin time (median 221 v 164 minutes, $p < 0.001$), longer warm-ischemia time (6 v 3 minutes, $p < 0.001$), less blood loss (100 v 240 ml, $p < 0.001$), and not a statistically different complication rate (intraoperatively 12% v 6%, $P = 0.49$, postoperatively both 6%). After laparoscopic nephrectomy, donors required less morphine (16 v 25 mg, $P = 0.005$) and shorter hospital stay (3 v 4 days, $P = 0.003$).[9] Lewis et al. performed a prospective study comparing traditional open, minimal-incision, and laparoscopic donor nephrectomy. They found median operating and first warm ischemia times that were longer for LDN than for MIDN (232vs147 min, $P < 0.001$; 2, 4 min, $P < 0.01$). Blood loss was not significantly higher for LDN (340 vs 260 ml). Hospital stay was significantly shorter for LDN (4.4 and 6 days), and postoperative morphine requirements were similar (71 vs 86, $P < 0.0001$), but the duration of the PCA was shorter(41, 53hours, $p<0.05$). Donors returned to work quicker after LDN than after MIDN (6vs 11vs 10; $P = 0.055$). [45]
The laparoscopic live donor nephrectomy is technically more demanding than the open approach, with a prolonged learning curve. Remarkably, the learning curve of the open approach was never described. Due to the learning curve, introduction of the laparoscopic method in small centers can be difficult and maybe other techniques are being preferred for safety reasons.

3.1.5 Transperitoneal versus retroperitoneal endoscopic donor nephrectomy

Transperitoneal and retroperitoneal donor nephrectomy can be practiced with or without hand-assistance. Endoscopic and hand-assisted trans- and retroperitoneal donornephrectomy are described above. Whether to take the retroperitoneal or the transperitoneal route for donor nephrectomy has not been solved yet. The limited retroperitoneal space makes it technically more challenging but provides superior access to posterior and particularly posteromedial space. Operative time is shorter in the transperitoneal group, and WIT tends to be longer. There is limited data confirming both techniques have equal complications, hospital stay, and graft and recipient survival.

3.1.6 Robotic-assisted donor nephrectomy

Robotic-assisted donor nephrectomy with the da Vinci robot can be performed with or without hand-assistance. The patient is placed in lateral decubitus position. Four trocars are used; two for the surgeon, a camera port and a port for the assistant. The surgeon is seated in a distant console. The images can be magnified and the movement of the articulated arm of the robot reproduces the action of the human wrist. An additional hand-assistance port in the midline can also be used. The nephrectomy is carried out in the same way as the laparoscopic procedure.

There are few articles on robot-assisted donor nephrectomy, but perhaps this will be expanded in this evolving field. Theoretical advantages of the robot-assisted technique are the combination of robotics and computer imaging, to enable microsurgery in a laparoscopic environment. There is one study comparing the robot-assisted donor nephrectomy (n=13) to the open donor nephrectomy (n=13). Renoult et al. found a longer operative- and warm ischemia time in the robot-assisted group (186 vs 113 min, $p<0.001$). There was no conversion in the robot-assisted group. There was one complication in both groups, a deep venous thrombosis in the robot-assisted group, and an acute pyelonephritis in the open group. Hospital stay was shorter after the RALD procedure (5.84+/-1.8 vs 9.69+/-2.2 days, $p<0.001$). Kidney function was equivalent for all donors, at 5 days and 1 month after nephrectomy. All kidneys started functioning immediately after the transplantation.[46]

	Level of evidence	Type of evidence
Conventional open VS mini-incision donor nephrectomy	III	- Prospective study - Retrospective studies, historical controls
Mini-incision VS laparoscopic donornephrectomy	I	- RCT - Prospective study - Meta-analysis
Laparoscopic VS hand-assisted laparoscopic donornephrectomy	II	- RCT - Prospective studies - Retrospective studies, historical controls
Laparoscopic VS hand-assisted retroperitoneal donornephrectomy	III	- Prospective - Retrospective
Robot-assisted VS open donor nephrectomy	III	- Retrospective, historical controls

Dols et al, Transpl Int. 2010 Feb;23(2):121-30.

Table 4. Operative techniques for live kidney donation; level and type of evidence.

3.2 Intra-operative complications

Intra-operative complications are important to note because of the high impact on donor and recipient life. There are not many studies describing the intra-operative complications as they are difficult to score uniformly. Only studies where a research fellow is present at the operation theater can give some information about the intra-operative complication rate. The rate of intra-operative complications is described in literature for the different techniques from 2 to 28% (table 5). There are no randomized studies reporting the intra-operative complications, as the inclusion number will be far too high.

Intra-operative complications are scored differently in all studies. Sorts of complications are: excessive blood loss, lesions to the small and large bowel, bladder, ureter and the kidney itself. We advocate a uniform system to score the complications by grade. The table below shows the modified Clavien scoring system, as we use for our intra- and postoperative complications (table 6).[47]

4. Post-operative

4.1 Outcome

Live kidney donation is relatively safe, but keeping in mind the otherwise healthy donor, it is never safe enough. Previous studies have shown that morbidity and mortality rates after LDN are low, with mortality estimated at 0.03%. Safety is gaining increasingly more interest and remains the big conundrum in minimal-invasive surgery. Safety consists of a few issues, not only the real complications but also the near complications or small intra and post-operative complications.

4.1.1 Long-term follow up

Adequate follow-up may identify donors who develop complications and to monitor the risks of life kidney donation. Donors who develop hypertension or a diminished kidney function may be identified and it may also aid donors from a social point of view. Some donors who struggle with their recovery or experience problems resuming work can be helped.

Literature indicates that the life expectancy of living kidney donors is similar to that of persons who have not donated a kidney. The risk of developing end-stage renal disease does not appear to be increased among kidney donors, and their current health seems to be similar to that of the general population. A lot of studies report on quality of life, and their quality of life appears to be very good. These outcomes may be a direct consequence of the meticulous routine screening of donors for important health conditions related to kidney disease at the time of donation.

After live kidney donation a reduction in total GFR of around 30% is described. This change in the GFR did not appear to increase over time. Kidney donation, or nephrectomy, is followed by a compensatory increase in the GFR in the remaining kidney to about 70% of pre nephrectomy values. The direct relationship between time since donation and the GFR may reflect not only a young age at donation but also the afore mentioned meticulous screening for underlying kidney disease that live kidney donors undergo. Compensatory hemodynamic changes in some animal models after a reduction of 50% or more in renal mass have been reported to be ultimately deleterious. There has been a concern that kidney donors might have damage in addition to the normal loss of kidney function with age.

	Intraoperative (%)	Postoperative (%)
Flank incision	2–13	8–35
MIDN	4–7	1–15
LDN	2.8–25	0–43
HALDN/HARP	4–28	0–15

Dols et al, Transpl Int. 2010 Feb;23(2):121-30.

Table 5. Intraoperative and postoperative complications (%) of the different types of operation techniques for live donor nephrectomy.

LDN	Grade*	Percentage of all complications (n = 10)	Percentage of total series (n= 40)	Complications	Patients (n)
	1	50 (n= 5)	12.5	Blood loss < 500 ml	5
	2	50 (n= 5)	3.8		5
	2a	10 (n= 1)	2.5	Blood loss >500 ml	1
	2b	30 (n= 3)	7.5	Small bowel injury	1
				Bladder lesion	1
				Ureteral injury	1
	2c	10 (n= 1)	2.5	No overview, conversion to hand-assisted LDN	1
	3	0	0	0	0
	4	0	0	0	0
HARP	**Grade***	**Percentage of all complications (n = 2)**	**Percentage of total series (n= 20)**	**Complications**	**Patients (n)**
	1	0	0	0	0
	2	100 (n= 2)	10	0	2
	2a	50 (n= 1)	5	Lumbar vein injury	1
	2b	0	0	0	0
	2c	50 (n= 1)	5	Lumbar vein injury, conversion	1
	3	0	0	0	0
	4	0	0	0	0

* 1 Non-life-threatening complications
2a Complications requiring only use of drug therapy, blood loss >500 mL or Hb drop >2 g/dL and/or resulting in hemodynamic instability or Hb <8 g/dL, readmission to hospital for medical management or prolongation of hospital stay for more than three times median length of stay.2b Complications requiring additional therapeutic intervention (ie operation for bowel obstruction, interventional radiologic procedure) or readmission to the hospital for intervention. 2c Complications requiring open conversion of LDN for patient management
3 Any complication with residual or lasting functional disability
4 Leads to renal failure or death in the donor

Dols et al, Transpl Int. 2010 Apr 1;23(4):358-63.

Table 6. Intraoperative complications of HARP and LDN with grading by severity.

Information regarding the long-term renal consequences of reduced renal mass in humans has come mainly from studies of children born with a reduced number of functioning nephrons, reports of focal sclerosis in patients with unilateral renal agenesis, and studies of World War II veterans who lost a kidney as a result of trauma. There are also numerous studies that have examined renal function in kidney donors. Although isolated cases of renal failure have been reported, no large study has shown evidence of progressive deterioration of renal function. Data suggests that there is no excess risk of ESRD in donors and confirms the view that factors linked to a reduced GFR in donors are the same as those that have been observed in the general population — namely, age and overweight. [3]
In previous studies the prevalence of hypertension and albuminuria in kidney donors were similar to those in controls who were matched for age, sex, race or ethnic group, and body-mass index, even two decades after donation.

5. Conclusion

Kidney transplantation is the therapy of choice for patients with end-stage renal disease and gives the best chance on long-term survival and a good quality of life. In the recent years there have been many changes in the living kidney donation programmes. Higher numbers of donors were operated due to less invasive surgical techniques, acceptable long-term safety and good transplant outcome. The surgical practice has evolved from the open lumbotomy, through mini-incision open donor nephrectomy (MIDN), to minimally invasive laparoscopic techniques. All different minimal invasive techniques, like standard laparoscopic, hand-assisted laparoscopic, hand-assisted retroperitoneoscopic and pure retroperitoneoscopic live donor nephrectomy, are practiced these days. Different centres have different visions on which technique to use, all depending on the expertise with each technique. In the literature there is Level I evidence that minimally invasive techniques are preferred above open, and mini-incision donor nephrectomy.
As LDN with or without hand-assistance has become the gold standard, the role for hand-assisted retroperitoneal and pure retroperitoneal donor nephrectomy requests further clarification. Outcome of most small, not randomized, studies comparing different minimal invasive techniques are similar in terms of intra- and post-operative outcome for donor and recipient.
Many centres in Europe implemented the LDN, but there are still a lot of centres where open donor nephrectomy is performed. For those centres that did not adopt the LDN, modified open or hand-assisted techniques may become a feasible alternative.
Safety of the laparoscopic technique is still debated, and the difficulty is that safety has never been studied as a primary endpoint because the sample size would be enormous. Therefore complications and conversions need to be registered in a national or international database.
The donor must be left with the best kidney and left as well as right may be selected for donation nowadays. Furthermore, donors having kidneys with multiple vessels and obese donors can be included if well-selected and offered proper follow-up. Future directions will have to focus on safety of surgical techniques, and long-term follow-up of live kidney donors and their recipients to guarantee a high standard of quality for the living related kidney donation programs.

6. References

[1] Kuss, R., J. Teinturier, and P. Milliez, *[Some attempts at kidney transplantation in man.].* Mem Acad Chir (Paris), 1951. 77(22-23-24): p. 755-64.

[2] Friedman, A.L., et al., *Fatal and Nonfatal Hemorrhagic Complications of Living Kidney Donation.* Ann Surg, 2006. 243(1): p. 126-130.
[3] Ibrahim, H.N., et al., *Long-term consequences of kidney donation.* N Engl J Med, 2009. 360(5): p. 459-69.
[4] Kok, N.F., et al., *Psychosocial and physical impairment after mini-incision open and laparoscopic donor nephrectomy: A prospective study.* Transplantation, 2006. 82(10): p. 1291-7.
[5] Kok, N.F., et al., *The current practice of live donor nephrectomy in europe.* Transplantation, 2006. 82(7): p. 892-7.
[6] Laupacis, A., et al., *A study of the quality of life and cost-utility of renal transplantation.* Kidney Int, 1996. 50(1): p. 235-42.
[7] Matas, A.J., et al., *2,500 living donor kidney transplants: a single-center experience.* Ann Surg, 2001. 234(2): p. 149-64.
[8] Liem, Y.S., et al., *Living renal donors: optimizing the imaging strategy--decision- and cost-effectiveness analysis.* Radiology, 2003. 226(1): p. 53-62.
[9] Kok, N.F., et al., *Comparison of laparoscopic and mini incision open donor nephrectomy: single blind, randomised controlled clinical trial.* BMJ, 2006. 333(7561): p. 221.
[10] Delmonico, F.L., *A Report of the Amsterdam Forum On the Care of the Live Kidney Donor: Data and Medical Guidelines.* Transplantation, 2005. 79(6 Suppl): p. S53-66.
[11] Gluecker, T.M., et al., *Comparison of CT angiography with MR angiography in the preoperative assessment of living kidney donors.* Transplantation, 2008. 86(9): p. 1249-56.
[12] Kok, N.F., et al., *Complex vascular anatomy in live kidney donation: imaging and consequences for clinical outcome.* Transplantation, 2008. 85(12): p. 1760-5.
[13] Mandal, A.K., et al., *Should the indications for laparascopic live donor nephrectomy of the right kidney be the same as for the open procedure? Anomalous left renal vasculature is not a contraindiction to laparoscopic left donor nephrectomy.* Transplantation, 2001. 71(5): p. 660-4.
[14] Abrahams, H.M., et al., *Technique, indications and outcomes of pure laparoscopic right donor nephrectomy.* J Urol, 2004. 171(5): p. 1793-6.
[15] Husted, T.L., et al., *Laparoscopic right living donor nephrectomy.* Transplant Proc, 2005. 37(2): p. 631-2.
[16] Kay, M.D., et al., *Comparison of right and left laparoscopic live donor nephrectomy.* BJU Int, 2006. 98(4): p. 843-4.
[17] Lind, M.Y., et al., *Right-sided laparoscopic live-donor nephrectomy: is reluctance still justified?* Transplantation, 2002. 74(7): p. 1045-8.
[18]Maciel, R.F., Hand-Assisted LaparoscopicLiveDonorNephrectomy(Right-Sided Approach): Experience Obtained From 31 Cases. Transplantation Proceedings, 2007. 39(8): p. 2476.
[19] Minnee, R.C., et al., *Left or right kidney in hand-assisted donor nephrectomy? A randomized controlled trial.* Transplantation, 2008. 85(2): p. 203-8.
[20] Narita, S., et al., *Outcome of right hand-assisted retroperitoneoscopic living donor nephrectomy.* Urology, 2006. 67(3): p. 496-500; discussion 500-1.
[21] Saad, S., et al., *Laparoscopic live donor nephrectomy for right kidneys: Experience in a German community hospital.* Surg Endosc, 2008. 22(3): p. 674-8.
[22] Desai, M.R., et al., Outcome of renal transplantation with multiple versus single renal arteries after laparoscopic live donor nephrectomy: a comparative study. Urology, 2007. 69(5): p. 824-7.
[23] Oh, H.K., A. Hawasli, and G. Cousins, *Management of renal allografts with multiple renal arteries resulting from laparoscopic living donor nephrectomy.* Clin Transplant, 2003. 17(4): p. 353-7.
[24] Saidi, R., et al., *Living donor kidney transplantation with multiple arteries: recent increase in modern era of laparoscopic donor nephrectomy.* Arch Surg, 2009. 144(5): p. 472-5.

[25] De La Vega, L.S., et al., *Patient and graft outcomes from older living kidney donors are similar to those from younger donors despite lower GFR.* Kidney Int, 2004. 66(4): p. 1654-61.

[26] Iordanous, Y., et al., *Recipient outcomes for expanded criteria living kidney donors: the disconnect between current evidence and practice.* Am J Transplant, 2009. 9(7): p. 1558-73.

[27] Johnson, S.R., et al., *Older living donors provide excellent quality kidneys: a single center experience (older living donors).* Clin Transplant, 2005. 19(5): p. 600-6.

[28] Kerr, S.R., et al., *Living donors >55 years: to use or not to use?* Transplantation, 1999. 67(7): p. 999-1004.

[29] Minnee, R.C., et al., *Older living kidney donors: surgical outcome and quality of life.* Transplantation, 2008. 86(2): p. 251-6.

[30] Naumovic, R., et al., *Effect of donor age on the outcome of living-related kidney transplantation.* Transpl Int, 2005. 18(11): p. 1266-74.

[31] Dols, L.F., et al., *Living kidney donors: impact of age on long-term safety.* Am J Transplant. 11(4): p. 737-42.

[32] Davis, C.L. and F.L. Delmonico, *Living-Donor Kidney Transplantation: A Review of the Current Practices for the Live Donor.* J Am Soc Nephrol, 2005. 16(7): p. 2098-2110.

[33] Heimbach, J.K., et al., *Obesity in living kidney donors: clinical characteristics and outcomes in the era of laparoscopic donor nephrectomy.* Am J Transplant, 2005. 5(5): p. 1057-64.

[34] Kok, N.F., et al., *Laparoscopic donor nephrectomy in obese donors: easier to implement in overweight women?* Transpl Int, 2007. 20(11): p. 956-61.

[35] Lynch, R.J., et al., *Obesity, surgical site infection, and outcome following renal transplantation.* Ann Surg, 2009. 250(6): p. 1014-20.

[36] Massarweh, N.N., et al., *High body mass index and short- and long-term renal allograft survival in adults.* Transplantation, 2005. 80(10): p. 1430-4.

[37] Srivastava, A., et al., *Subcostal versus transcostal mini donor nephrectomy: is rib resection responsible for pain related donor morbidity.* J Urol, 2003. 170(3): p. 738-40.

[38] Kok, N.F., et al., *Mini-incision open donor nephrectomy as an alternative to classic lumbotomy: evolution of the open approach.* Transpl Int, 2006. 19(6): p. 500-5.

[39] Neipp, M., et al., *Living donor nephrectomy: flank incision versus anterior vertical mini-incision.* Transplantation, 2004. 78(9): p. 1356-61.

[40] Bargman, V., et al., *Randomized trial of laparoscopic donor nephrectomy with and without hand assistance.* J Endourol, 2006. 20(10): p. 717-22.

[41] Gjertsen, H., et al., *Introduction of hand-assisted retroperitoneoscopic living donor nephrectomy at Karolinska University Hospital Huddinge.* Transplant Proc, 2006. 38(8): p. 2644-5.

[42] Sundqvist, P., et al., *Hand-assisted retroperitoneoscopic live donor nephrectomy in comparison to open and laparoscopic procedures: a prospective study on donor morbidity and kidney function.* Transplantation, 2004. 78(1): p. 147-53.

[43] Wadstrom, J., P. Lindstrom, and B.M. Engstrom, *Hand-assisted retroperitoneoscopic living donor nephrectomy superior to laparoscopic nephrectomy.* Transplant Proc, 2003. 35(2): p. 782-3.

[44] Leventhal, J.R., et al., *Laparoscopic donor nephrectomy 1997 to 2003: lessons learned with 500 cases at a single institution.* Surgery, 2004. 136(4): p. 881-90.

[45] Lewis, G.R., et al., *A comparison of traditional open, minimal-incision donor nephrectomy and laparoscopic donor nephrectomy.* Transpl Int, 2004. 17(10): p. 589-95.

[46] Renoult, E., et al., *Robot-assisted laparoscopic and open live-donor nephrectomy: a comparison of donor morbidity and early renal allograft outcomes.* Nephrol Dial Transplant, 2006. 21(2): p. 472-7.

[47] Kocak, B., et al., *Proposed classification of complications after live donor nephrectomy.* Urology, 2006. 67(5): p. 927-31.

5

The Role of Laparoscopy in the Management of End-Stage Renal Disease Patients in Peritoneal Dialysis

Rui Maio
Universidade de Lisboa
Portugal

1. Introduction

Continuous ambulatory peritoneal dialysis (CAPD) is an established and well-known technique for renal replacement therapy in patients with end-stage renal disease (1,2). Since the introduction of CAPD, four methods have been advocated for the placement of PD catheters: open surgery, percutaneous, peritoneoscopic (Y-Tec; Medigroup, Oswego, Illinois, USA), and laparoscopic placement (2,3,13,17).

The manner in which PD catheters are placed has a significant influence on catheter function, incidence of catheter-related complications, and technique survival (6). Open surgery and especially the percutaneous technique are associated with poor outcomes and sometimes life-threatening complications (20,21). In fact, the incidence of omental wrapping, catheter displacement, and intraabdominal complications, specifically bowel and bladder perforation, is higher with these two methods. In recent years, there has been considerable interest in the use of laparoscopy for creation of peritoneal access. Laparoscopic peritoneal catheter placement is simple, quick, efficient, and minimally invasive. As with any new application of a modality, laparoscopy for peritoneal access is still undergoing procedure-specific adaptation. The strength of laparoscopy is that it allows an opportunity to visibly address problems that adversely effect catheter outcome, namely, catheter tip migration, omental entrapment, and peritoneal adhesions. Identifying and preemptively correcting these problems at the time of the implantation procedure are the advantages of surgical laparoscopy over other catheter insertion techniques (7,8).

Regardless of the technique utilized to implant the PD catheter, there are best-demonstrated practices that should be followed in every case (4,5). Adherence to these recognized practices could reduce the risk of catheter tip migration, pericatheter leakage, hernias, superficial cuff extrusion, and catheter-related infections.

2. Laparoscopic placement of Tenckhoff catheters: A safe, effective, and reproducible procedure

Our catheter implantation technique will be described in detail (14,15,16).

The same team operated on all patients. The laparoscopic procedures were performed in the operating room under general anesthesia. A prophylactic antibiotic, cefazolin – or vancomycin in the event of cephalosporin allergy – was administered prior to the procedure. A Veress needle was inserted into the peritoneal cavity through a stab incision in the right hypochondrium to create a pneumoperitoneum. Pressure limits for abdominal gas insufflation were set between 10 and 12 mmHg. The Veress needle was replaced with a 10-mm port and preliminary laparoscopy was performed to look for adhesions or other anatomical abnormalities that could hinder performance of the Tenckhoff catheter. A 5-mm port was inserted under direct vision in the right iliac fossa. A 1-cm skin incision was made on the left, 2 - 3 cm lateral and inferior to the umbilicus, and a second 5-mm port was placed in a paramedian location and tunneled in a caudal direction through the rectus sheath for a distance of at least 4 cm before entry was made into the peritoneal cavity. We aligned both 5-mm ports and inserted the Endograsp (United States Surgical, Norwalk, Connecticut, USA) through the lower right quadrant port and brought it out through the paramedian port. The paramedian port was then removed but the tip of the Endograsp remained outside the abdominal cavity (Figures 1 and 2). The intraperitoneal portion of the Tenckhoff catheter tip was caught with the grasper and slowly pulled inside the peritoneal cavity through the tunnel created in the abdominal wall (Figure 3). The deep cuff was located at the medial edge of the muscle within the rectus sheath. The intra-abdominal portion of the catheter was placed between the visceral and parietal peritoneum toward the pouch of Douglas. The subcutaneous tunnel tract and skin exit site were directed downwards or laterally. The subcutaneous cuff was positioned at a distance of at least 2 cm from the exit wound. Between each of the preceding steps, catheter patency was checked to ensure that there was adequate inflow and outflow without leakage. The entire procedure was done under direct vision. The laparoscope was then removed and the pneumoperitoneum was allowed to deflate. The fascia of the laparoscopic port site was closed with 2-0 polyglactin suture. Skin wounds were sutured with 3-0 nylon. The protocol for catheter irrigation consisted of a daily in-and-out flush with dialysate solution. Peritoneal dialysis was generally delayed for a minimum of 2 weeks to allow complete wound healing.

Since January 2002, the author performed more then 400 laparoscopic placement of Tenckhoff peritoneal catheter in patients with end-stage renal diseases.

The average operative time was 15 ± 4 minutes and mean duration of hospital stay was 1 day. There were no conversions from laparoscopy to any other conventional method of catheter placement. In patients with intraperitoneal adhesions, laparoscopic adhesiolysis was performed to eliminate intraperitoneal loculations that might interfere with the peritoneal catheter drainage function.

No infections of the exit site or subcutaneous tunnel, hemorrhagic complications, abdominal wall hernias, or extrusion of the superficial catheter cuff were detected.

No mortality occurred in this series of patients. Catheter survival was 97%, 95%, and 91% at 1, 2, and 3 years, respectively (Figure 4).

Peritoneal catheter placement must be regarded as an important surgical intervention, demanding care and attention to detail equal to that of any other surgical procedure and as a consequence a competent and experienced operator must perform the catheter implantation procedure.

Due to its characteristics (simple, quick, efficient, and minimally invasive to the patient), it seems that laparoscopic peritoneal catheter placement should become the preferred approach. In addition, the laparoscopic method offers an excellent view of the abdomen and optimal placement of the catheter within the cavity. The single blind step is the Veress needle insertion; however, the probability of damaging the abdominal organs or epigastric and retroperitoneal blood vessels is very low.

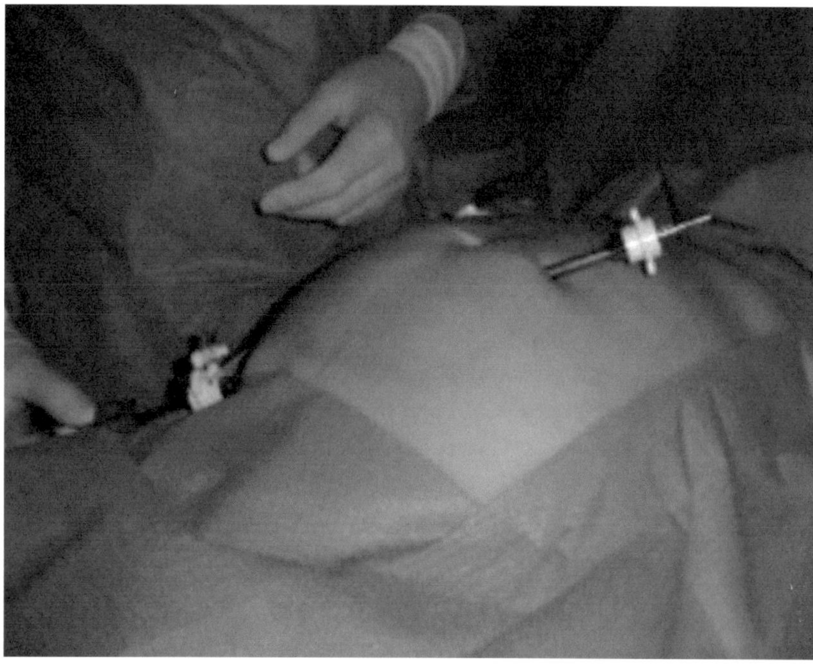

Fig. 1. Operative photograph demonstrates the alignment of the two 5-mm ports and insertion of the grasping forceps.

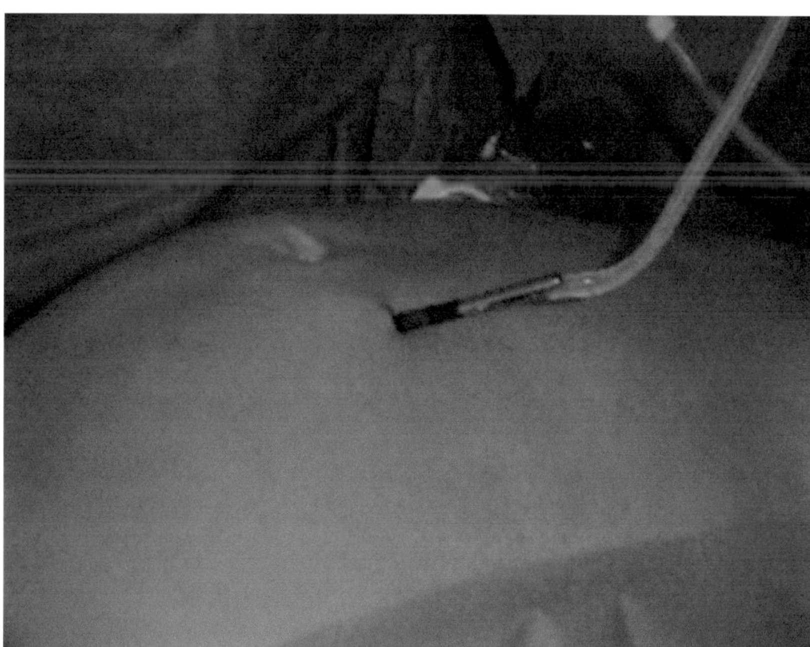

Fig. 2. Operative photograph shows that the tunneled5-mm port has been removed and the dialysis catheter has been grasped in preparation of pulling it into the peritoneal cavity.

This method is particularly useful in patients that have already undergone previous abdominal operations (8). Patients with peritoneal adhesions that might interfere with drainage function can be treated with adhesiolysis and displaced catheters can be repositioned.
In addition, laparoscopy is useful for the diagnosis and treatment of abdominal wall hernias and peritoneo- vaginal canal persistence.
Another advantage of laparoscopy is the possibility of performing a selective prophylactic omentopexy, a technique that has been separately described by Ogunc and Crabtree (10,11). In conjunction with rectus sheath tunneling and adhesiolysis, it is possible that selective use of omentopexy could have prevented the omental obstruction and the need for revisionary surgery that occurred in 6 of our patients.
Some centers use laparoscopic insertion with local anesthesia on the assumption that it is safer (12). We suggest that modern general anesthesia is safe for the vast majority of patients and allows a better view of the peritoneal cavity. Different techniques have been described for the placement of peritoneal catheters by laparoscopy using specially designed devices. The distinctive characteristic of our technique is that we used nothing more than conventional laparoscopic equipment available in any facility that routinely performs laparoscopic surgery. Laparoscopy is a commonly performed procedure in general practice but it also has an inherently steep learning curve. A junior surgeon, under close supervision of a consultant, performed some of the later procedures without technical difficulties.

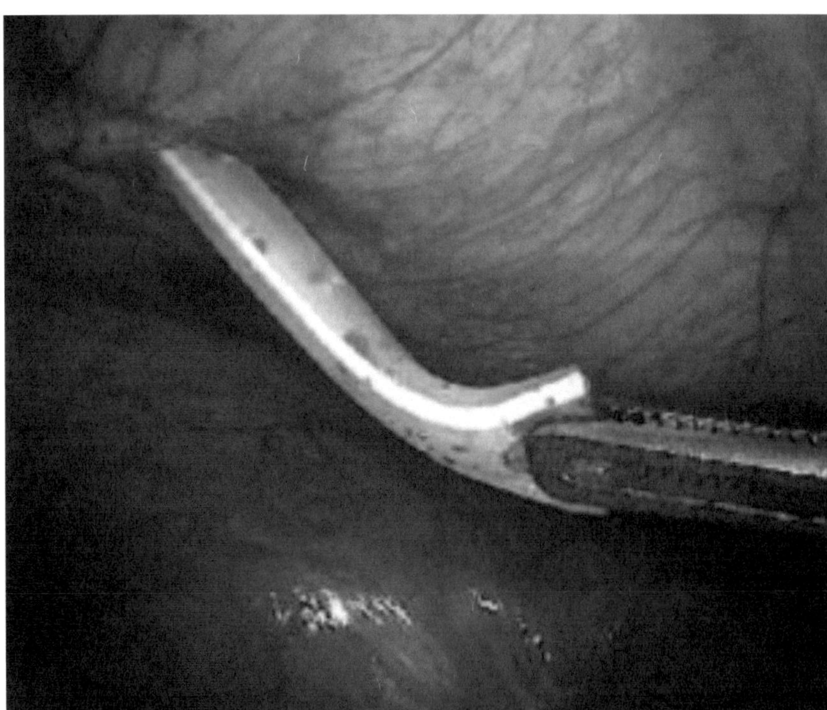

Fig. 3. Operative photograph shows the catheter tip pulled inside the peritoneum through the tunnel created in the abdominal wall.

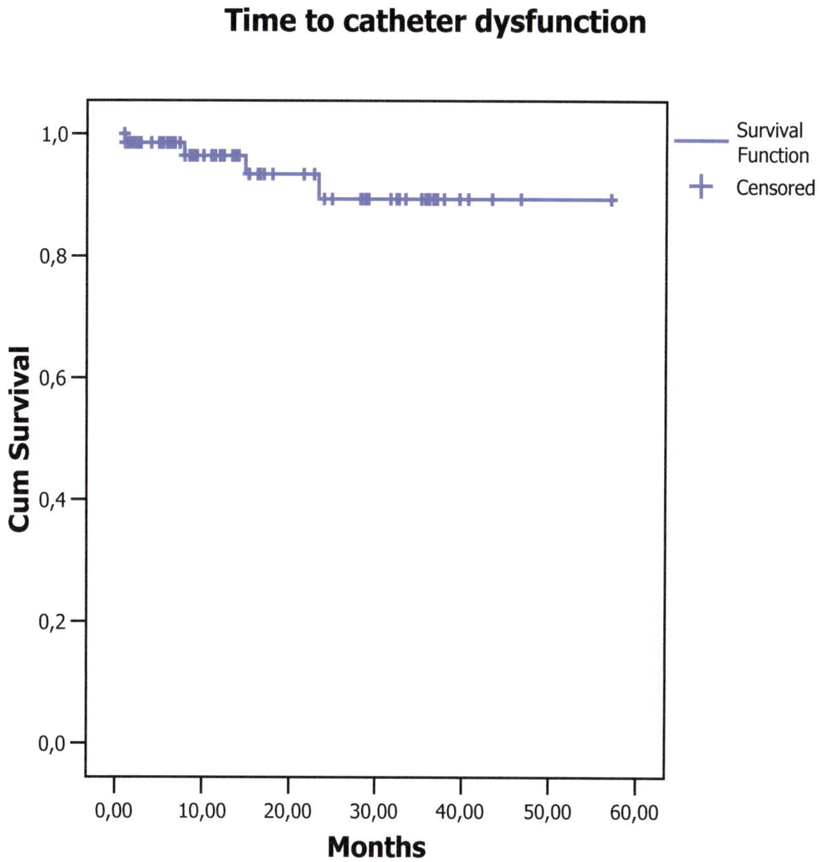

Fig. 4. Cumulative probability of peritoneal dialysis catheter survival following laparoscopic placement. The ticks on the survival curve represent censored data points.

Abdominal wall leaks, our major complication occurred at the beginning of our experience. At that time, the length of the musculofascial tunnel was shorter and in our opinion resulted in a higher incidence of leaks. Successful management of these leaks consisted of delaying the beginning of dialysis.

We did not experience intraoperative complications such as intra-abdominal organ injury, as has been reported for conventional techniques. In fact, in our series we had no intra-abdominal catastrophes and the incidence of catheter displacement was lower than that reported using open surgery technique. Furthermore, we did not encounter problems commonly reported for open catheter placement, such as hematoma, seroma, or infections. No perioperative mortality occurred in this case series. Our long-term catheter survival exceeds the targets recommended by published guidelines and is higher than most reported experiences.

3. Abdominal adhesions

Despite widespread acceptance of peritoneal dialysis, patients with previous history of abdominal operations are frequently excluded from consideration.

Abdominal surgery can lead to the formation of adhesions. Adhesive scarring within the peritoneal space can complicate catheter placement. Compartmentalization of the peritoneal cavity by adhesions can impede insertion of the catheter, produce kinking or malpositioning of the tubing, block the side drainage holes resulting in flow dysfunction, and limit the available dialyzable space. It is not unreasonable to surmise that intraperitoneal adhesions would not only increase the difficulty and risk of catheter insertion but also adversely affect catheter survival.

Peritoneal adhesions have been reported to form after 70-90% of abdominal operations. Catheter implantation using conventional approaches in patients with intra-abdominal adhesions has been associated with an increased incidence of postoperative complications. In the presence of adhesions, catheter insertion can be complicated by visceral injury, hemorrhage and catheter malposition with flow dysfunction. Visualization of peritoneal cavity during implantation of PD catheters using laparoscopic methods can determine the presence and extent of intra-abdominal adhesions and help direct the placement of catheters. Patients with peritoneal adhesions that might interfere with drainage function can be treated with adhesiolysis and displaced catheters can be repositioned. Therefore this method is particularly useful in patients that have already undergone previous abdominal operations.

4. Omental wrap

Omental wrap is a common cause of catheter obstruction. The mechanism of omental wrap is uncertain. A redundant omentum can adhere to the distal end of the catheter and displace it out of the pelvis. A catheter that has migrated out of the pelvis is at risk of being wrapped by the omentum. Catheter displacement as seen on plain abdominal radiograph could in fact be omental wrap.

Laparoscopic intervention is an effective treatment for omental wrap. The tiny projections of the omentum insinuate through the side holes of the catheter and obstruct its lumen. On close-up view, the omental fat forms a dumb-bell shaped plug in the side hole. The plug is snug and firm. While the catheter is being steadied by laparoscopic graspers, the omental plugs have to be pulled in the right direction to be released. A less precise manoeuvre, such as pulling the catheter away from the omentum, is unlikely to free the catheter entirely, and bleeding might occur as the omental plugs together with the small vessels supplying them are avulsed. This can happen in fluoroscopic stiff-wire manipulation, since the movement involved is similar. Reports of stiff wire manipulation under fluoroscopic guidance showed a high incidence of recurrent malfunction and the need for repeat manipulation.

Omental wrap remains one of the likely reasons for failure of non-laparoscopic treatments. In one study, 50% of the patients who had undergone unsuccessful fluoroscopic wire manipulation were found to have omental wrap at laparoscopic salvage. One definitive laparoscopic procedure is likely to be more effective than multiple wire manipulations. For recurrent catheter migration or malfunction, laparoscopy should be the next step. Open removal and replacement of catheter risks recurrent malfunction since the cause of malfunction has not been resolved.

Laparoscopy provides visual diagnosis of the cause of catheter malfunction and when used as first-line management, has shown high success rates.

A procedure on the greater omentum appears important in preventing catheter malfunction. A low rate of obstruction has been demonstrated by series of primary open insertion of catheter where prophylactic omentopexy or subtotal omentectomy had been performed. Crabtree and Fishman reported an obstruction rate of only 0.7% in 153 patients when selective prophylactic omentopexy during laparoscopic implantation of catheter was performed. Reports of laparoscopic salvage have found an incidence of omental wrap ranging from 57 to 92%. The incidence of obstruction causing poor flow of dialysate is 6.0 to 20.5%. Occlusion by the greater omentum is therefore an important etiology of catheter malfunction. Current laparoscopic techniques for salvaging catheters include simple repositioning with or without catheter fixation, omentopexy, omentectomy and omental folding.

Omentopexy is a laparoscopically enabled procedure shown to be of value in preventing omental entrapment. Ogunc recommended it for all implantation procedures whereas Crabtree *et al* used it selectively when redundant omentum was found to extend to the deep pelvis in the vicinity of the catheter tip. In Ogunc' s Technique which is minilaparoscopic extraperitoneal tunelling with omentopexy, the lateral inferior edges of the omentum are fixed onto the parietal peritoneum of the lateral abdominal wall at two points with a 3-0 polypropylene suture with 2 mm needle holder at the level of the umbilicus (18). If the omentum is large or bulky, one more fixation suture is applied between the middle inferior edge of the omentum and the falciform ligament. There was no complication related to the small bowel volvulus, internal herniation and the other mechanical outflow obstruction in 44 consecutive patients.

In contrast to omentopexy, which fixes the omentum to the anterior or lateral abdominal wall, or to the falciform ligament, omental folding fixes the omentum to itself. Omental folding creates a safe distance between the catheter and the omentum by shortening the latter. Technically, omental folding is a form of omentopexy. The other effect of folding is that the distal omentum with its slender projections is converted into a rounded edge.

Omental folding can thus be performed with the most basic laparoscopic equipment found in most surgical units. With practice, the folding of the omentum can be performed within 10 minutes and the whole salvage procedure can take less than 40 minutes and is a safe and effective technique for salvaging PD catheters (19).

5. Conclusions

A laparoscopic approach for placing Tenckhoff catheters can be accomplished with complete compliance to recommended best practices for PD access. Moreover, laparoscopy permits advantages over conventional implantation techniques through the use of adjunctive procedures such as rectus sheath tunneling to prevent catheter tip migration, adhesiolysis to assure adequate dialysate drainage function of the catheter, and omentopexy, omentectomy or omental folding to prevent omental wrapping. The catheter implantation method described in this chapter uses standard laparoscopic equipment and techniques completely familiar to any surgeon who routinely performs laparoscopic surgery. The procedure can be performed with low risks of morbidity and mortality. The patient benefits from a minimally invasive approach and the assurance of obtaining successful long-term catheter function. The results reported here support our opinion that laparoscopic Tenckhoff catheter implantation should become the standard of care for clinical practice.

6. References

[1] Gokal R. CAPD overview. Perit Dial Int 1996; 16(Suppl 1):13-18.

[2] Cruz C. Implantation techniques for peritoneal dialysis catheters. Perit Dial Int 1996; 16(Suppl 1):319–21.
[3] Gokal R, Alexander S, Ash SR, Chen TW, Danielson A, Holmes C, et al. Peritoneal catheters and exit-site practices toward optimum peritoneal access: 1998 update. Perit Dial Int 1998; 18:11–33.
[4] Dombros N, Dratwa M, Feriani M, Gokal R, Heimburger O, Krediet R, et al.; EBPG-Expert Group on Peritoneal Dialysis. European best practice guidelines for peritoneal dialysis. . Nephrol Dial Transplant 2005; 20:ix8–12.
[5] Lund L. Per itoneal dialysis catheter placement: is laparoscopy an option? Int Urol Nephrol 2007; 39:625–8.
[6] Asif A. Peritoneal dialysis catheter insertion. Minerva Chir 2005; 60:417–28.
[7] Adamson AS. Endoscopic placement of CAPD catheters: an overview of one hundred procedures. Nephrol Dial Transplant 1992; 7:855–7.
[8] Brandt CP. Laparoscopic placement of peritoneal dialysis catheters in patients who have undergone prior abdominal operations. J Am Coll Surg 1994; 178:515–16.
[9] Kimmelstiel FM. Laparoscopic management of peritoneal dialysis catheters. Surg Gynecol Obstet 1993; 176:565–70.
[10] Ogunc G. Videolaparoscopy with omentopexy: a new technique to allow placement of a catheter for continuous ambulatory peritoneal dialysis. Surg Today 2001; 31: 942–4.
[11] Crabtree JH, Fishman A. Selective performance of prophylactic omentopexy during laparoscopic implantation of peritoneal dialysis catheters. Surg Laparosc Endosc Percutan Tech 2003; 13:180–4.
[12] Crabtree JH. Laparoscopic approach under local anesthesia for peritoneal dialysis access. Perit Dial Int 2000; 20: 757–65.
[13] Cala Z. Laparoscopic placement of the peritoneal dialysis catheter using a specially designed trocar: a review of 84 patients. Dial Transplant 2000; 11:722 7.
[14] Maio R. Colocação de cateteres de diálise peritoneal. Método cirúrgico-vantagens e inconvenientes. III curso pós-graduado de diálise peritoneal. Lisboa; 2005.
[15] Maio R. Laparoscopic placement of peritoneal dialysis catheter—single centre experience. 7th European Peritoneal Dialysis Meeting; October 15-18, 2005; Prague, Czech Republic.
[16] Maio et al. Laparoscopic placement of Tenckhoff catheters for peritoneal dialysis: a safe, effective and reproducible procedure. Perit Dial Int 2008; 28:170-3.
[17] Poole et al. Laparoscopic Tenckhoff catheter insertion: a prospective study of a new technique. Aust NZ J Surg 2000; 70:371-3.
[18] Ogunc. Minilaparoscopic extraperitoneal tunneling with omentopexy: a new technique for CAPD catheter placement. Perit Dial Int 2005; 25:551-5.
[19] Comert et al. A new laparoscopic technique for the placement of a permanent peritoneal dialysis catheter: the preperitoneal tunneling method. Surg Endosc 2005; 19:245-248.
[20] Soontrapornchai et al. Comparison of open and laparoscopic secure placement of peritoneal dialysis catheters. Surg Endosc 2005; 19:137-9.
[21] Jwo SC et al. Prospective randomized study for comparison of open surgery with laparoscopic-assisted placement of Tenckhoff peritoneal dialysis catheter--a single center experience and literature review. J Surg Res. 2010 Mar;159(1):489-96. Epub 2008 Oct 9

6

Laparoscopic Extraperitoneal Approach for Urinary Bladder Stones Removal – A New Operative Technique

Tsvetin Genadiev
University Hospital Lozenetz
Bulgaria

1. Introduction

The classical operative treatment methods of urinary bladder stones are open suprapubic operation or transurethral lithotripsy. Alternative methods are suprapubic endoscopic extraction of bladder stones and combined transurethral and suprapubic technique. In the present work we describe a novel endoscopic method for urinary bladder stones removal. The urethral trauma is the main reason against the transurethral access for large or multiple bladder stones.

After the pub med investigation according to the key words laparoscopy, endoscopic extraction bladder stones, retroperitoneoscopic urinary bladder stones removal, endoscopic sectio alta, there are no results similar to our technique.

To the best of our knowledge, this is the first description of this technique. This novel method we named Endoscopic Sectio Alta - ESAL.

1.1 History of urinary bladder stones treatment

The bladder stones are about 5% of all urinary stones. The forming reasons are urinary infection, corpus alienum in bladder, obstruction or previous prostatic operation (Schwartz BF& Stoller ML, 2000).

According to Ellis H. 1979 the first surgical operation to remove bladder stones is perineal lithotomy described by Aulus Celsus in first century AD. In 1561, Pierre Franco made suprapubic vesicotomy - the so called High operation. In 1719 John Douglas, a brother of the famous surgeon James Douglas, described surgical technique based on opening the bladder after filling it with water without opening the peritoneum. This procedure made the High operation even more popular (H. Ellis, 1979). The open technique is currently applied successfully on aged patients and children (Chow & Chou, 2008). Nowadays the progress in medical techniques and technology has lead to a number of endoscopic methods such as transurethral lithotomy, percutaneous suprapubic cystolithotripsy and a combination of both methods - transurethral and percutaneous (Holman et al., 2004; Tugcu et al.; 2009 Wollin et al., 1994).

2. Operative technique

2.1 Patient selection

The patient selection for ESAL is based on the number and the size of the stones. Suitable for ESAL are patients with single large (more than three centimeters) bladder stone, without residual urine. Usually those are the stones, which have migrated from the kidney. Another group of appropriate candidates are patients with multiple (more than five) bladder stones with size ranging between one and two centimeters. There were no uric acid stones treated in this study.

2.2 Patients

Five male patients, all of which having urinary bladder stones and aged between 52 and 58 years underwent Endoscopic Sectio Alta in our clinic. One of the cases is with a single 4 centimeters large stone and the others are with multiple four to five stones with sizes between 1 and 1.5 centimeters. All stones were x-ray positive. The patients underwent abdominal ultrasound of the urinary bladder and plain x-ray film on kidney, ureter and bladder (KUB). Middle prostatic size was 45 cubic centimeters on the abdominal ultrasound. There were no cases with residual urine. All patients wanted prostate spearing methods and were informed and agreed with our technique.

2.3 Contraindications

The contraindications to ESAL are those conditions that are contradictory to any laparoscopy, such as severe haemostatic disorder or cardiopulmonary disease. Patients with previous operations such as inguinal hernioplasty or appendectomy are not contraindicated. Patients after open urinary bladder surgery for prostatic adenomectomy or for another reason have relatively contraindicated for ESAL.

2.4 Preoperative preparation

The patients were given laxative suppository in the evening before operative day and again 2 hours before operation. Suprapubic area was shaved up to the umbilicus and compressive stockings were placed on the legs.

2.5 Anesthesia

General endotracheal anesthesia is usually preferable for laparoscopy. This anesthesia was used in all cases.

2.6 Intraoperative patient preparation

The patient is in the horizontal supine position with shoulders support for Trendelenburg position. The legs are in slight abduction. A nasogastric tube is not necessary because of the short operative time and the extraperitoneal access. The Foley catheter is placed in a sterile fashion after the draping was completed.

2.7 Operative team

The operative team consists of a surgeon, an assistant and a nurse. The surgeon stands on the patient's left side while the assistant stands on the patient's right side. A laparoscopic tower and a single monitor are placed between the patient's legs.

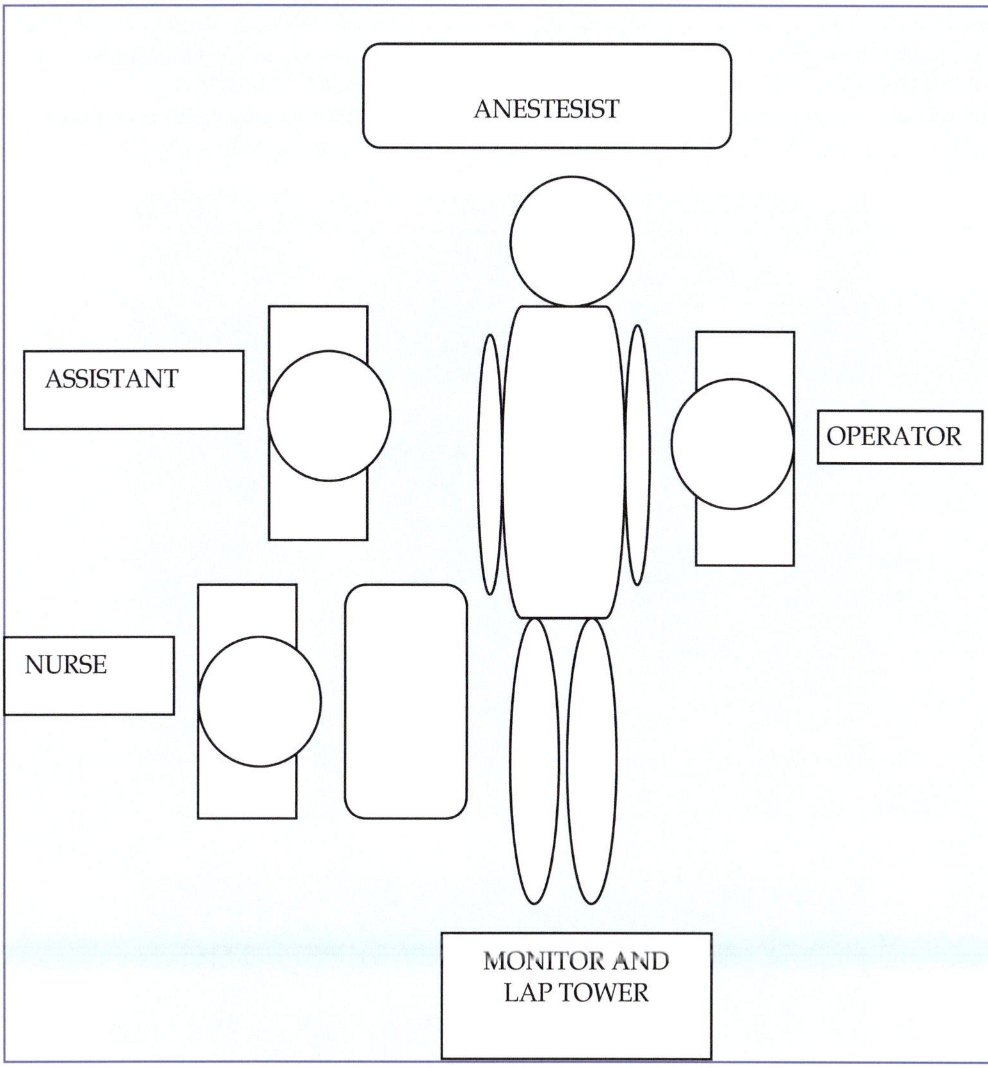

Fig. 1. Schematic of the operative team placement.

2.8 Instruments

We used the standard equipment for laparoscopic operation comprised of monitor, insufflator, electrosurgical monopolar and bipolar device, suction-irrigation device, xenon light source, and 10 mm, 0-degree lens laparoscope. Four trocars were placed - two of them were 10 mm long and were used for a camera and the operator, two were 5 mm long for the operator and one were 5 mm long for the assistant. Bipolar and monopolar dissectors, monopolar scissors, suction-irrigation canula, needleholders, endobag were also employed.

3. Primary access

The operation started with retroperitoneoscopic praeperitoneal and praevesical space made following the Endoscopic Extraperitoneal Radical Prostatectomy (EERPE) technique,

described by J-U Stolzenburg (Stolzenburg JU, 2002). The operative access started with a 2 centimeters wide periumbilical skin incision above right musculus rectus abdominis - figure 2. After that, the anterior rectus fascia was transversally incised - figure 3.
The balloon trocar was insufflated carefully and gradually with a small volume of CO_2 until the anterior abdominal wall became slightly prominent above the umbilicus level.

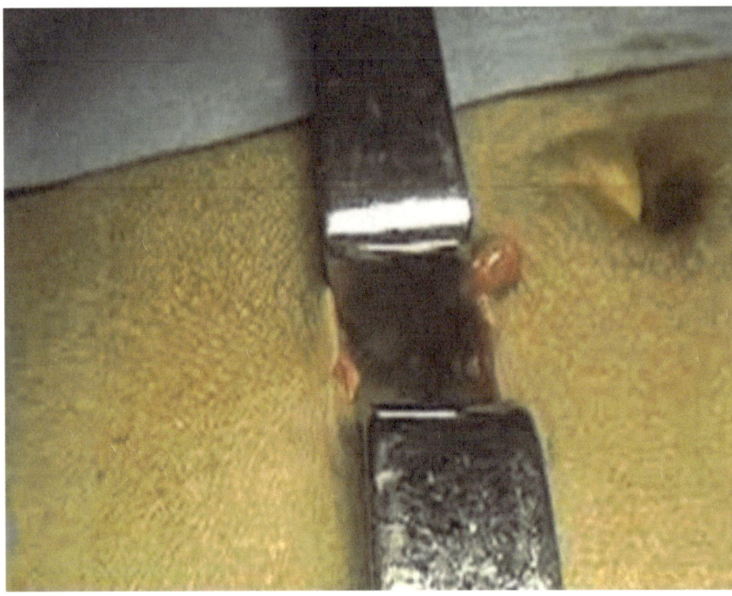

Fig. 2. Periumbilical skin incision above the right musculus rectus abdominis

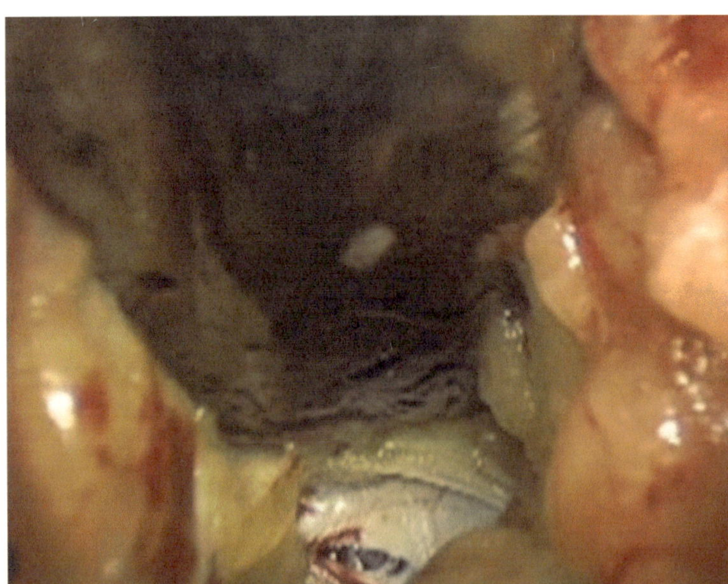

Fig. 3. The picture shows transversal incision of the anterior rectus fascia.

Attention should be paid not to damage the vasa epigastria.
Two lateral sutures of the rectus fascia were made in other to keep in place the conical camera trocar.

3.1 Trocar placement

Trocar placement was similar to the endoscopic extraperitoneal access only without the second trocar in the right side.
The camera trocar was with conical shape, 10-mm in size and was placed on the paraumbilical right side. On the left side lateral of the patient was placed 10-mm trocar and a medial 5-mm trocar. On the assistant side there was only one 5-mm trocar - figure 4.

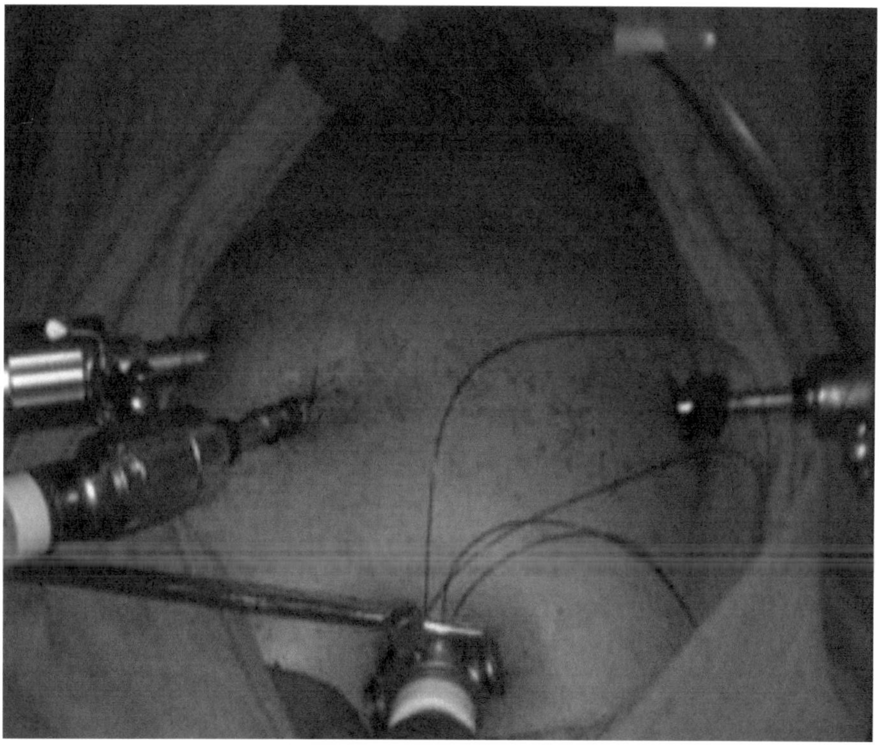

Fig. 4. The picture shows trocar placement - 10-mm conical camera trocar, fixed with fascial sutures. At the left side lateral there is a 10-mm trocar and the medial is 5-mm. At the right side there is one 5-mm trocar.

3.2 Operative technique

The working CO_2 pressure was between 12 and 14 mmHg. The urinary bladder was inflated with 150 milliliters saline water to locate its front side. The anterior bladder wall was laterally sutured with two 2/0 stitches in a distance of about 3 to 4 centimeters and was lifted - as shown on figure 5. Vesicotomy was performed at two centimeters between the stitches with monopolar scissors - figure 6. The bladder was inspected for damages and residual stones - figure 7.

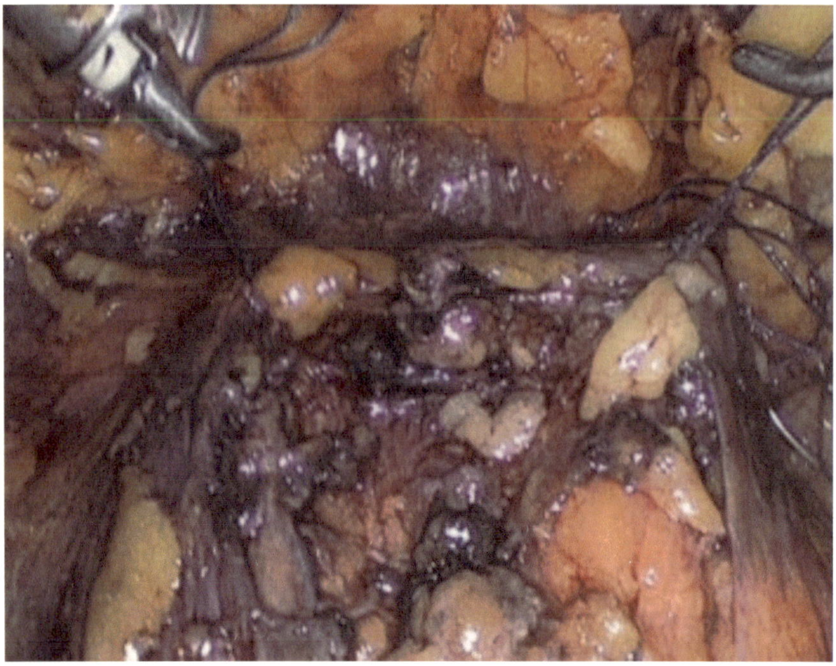

Fig. 5. The picture shows the anterior lateral bladder wall sutured with two 2/0 stitches. Retzius space remains closed for minimally operative trauma and against stone migration.

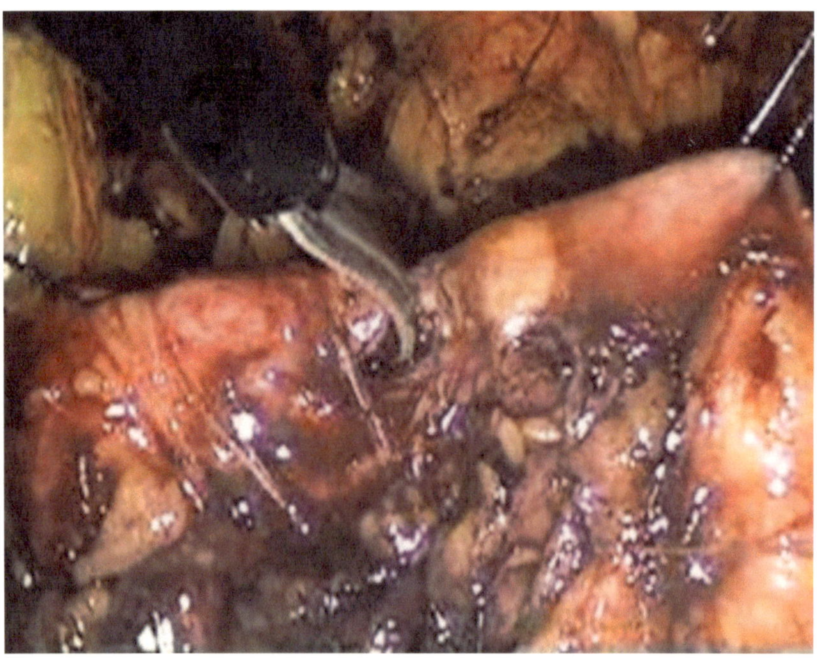

Fig. 6. The picture shows vesicotomy perfomed at 2 centimeters between the stitches with monopolar scissors.

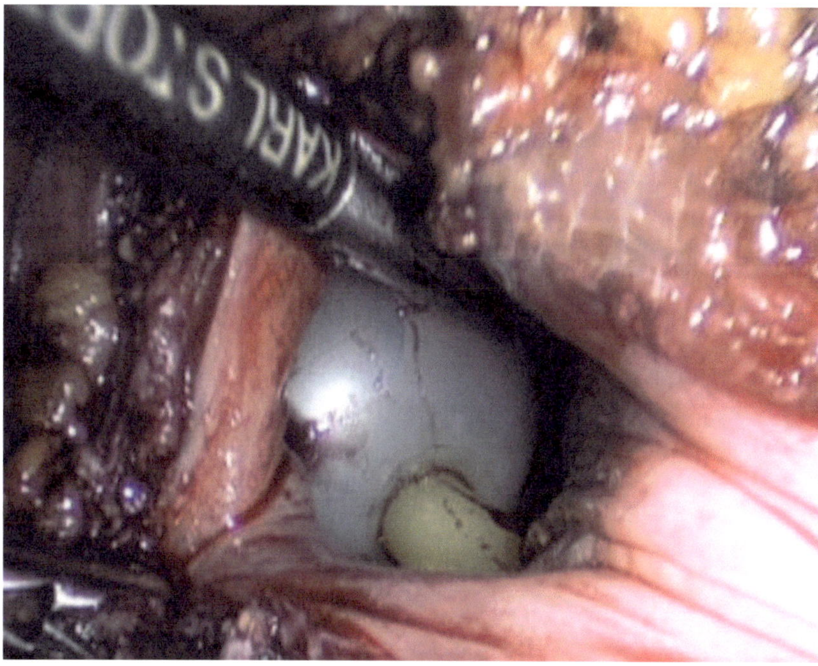

Fig. 7. The picture shows inspection inside bladder.

After the bladder inspection, the stones were extracted and put into the endobag - figure 8.

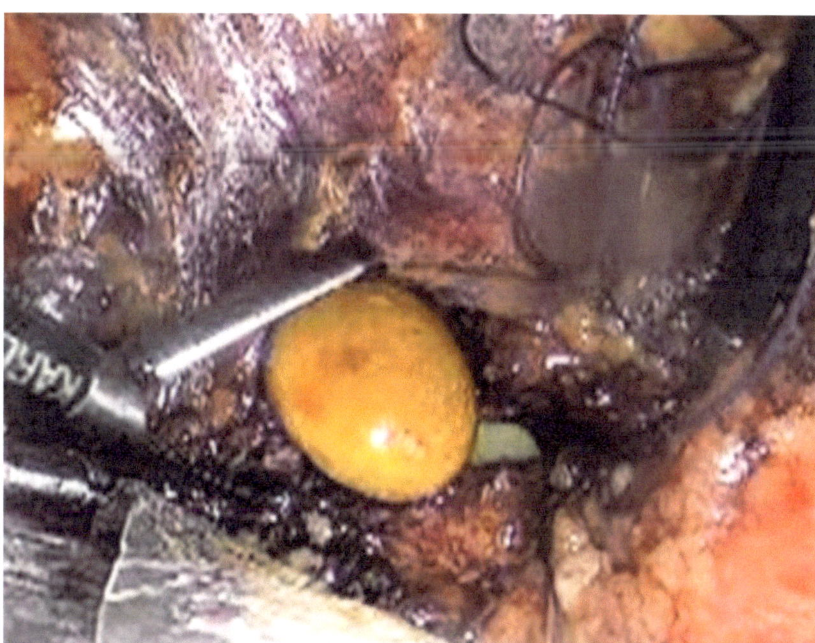

Fig. 8. The picture shows the extraction of the stones and put them into the endobag.

The bladder wall is sutured with running suture 2/0 resorbable suture - figure 9.

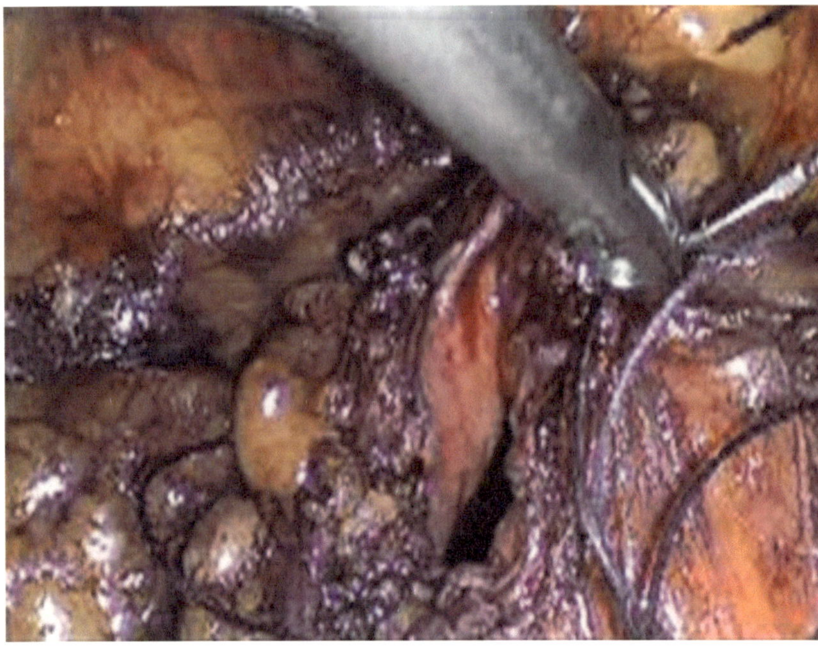

Fig. 9. The picture shows closure the bladder wall with running suture 2/0 resorbable suture.

The endobag was extracted through the camera port. Praevesical tube drainage was placed for 24 hours. The fascia at the camera port and the skin incisions were closed.

3.3 Postoperative care and results

Prophylactic with a third generation cephalosporin and low molecular heparin was usually performed. The Foley catheter was kept in place for 3 days. There was no postoperative severe pain. The drainage was kept until second postoperative day. The patients were able to move and drink water in several hours after the operation. Hospital stay was between 3 and 4 days. There were no cases of conversion or operative revision.

3.4 Complications

There were no major intraoperative or postoperative complications. In one case during the operation, we performed cystoscopy because of the smal number of extracted stones. On the postoperative x-ray plain film, was registered one stone, which has probably migrated outside the bladder. One month later, the patient was in good condition, without stones in the urinary bladder. One year later the same patient has two stones in the urinary bladder. We offered him a second operation - transurethral stones lithotripsy and prostate resection. There is one case of subcutaneous hematomas probably due to of early drainage removing - figure 10.

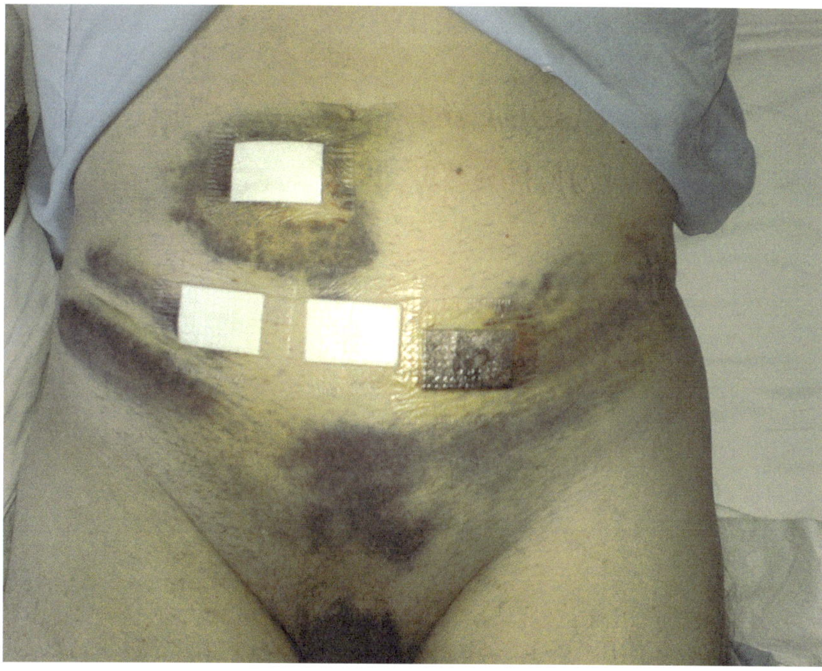

Fig. 10. The picture shows the patient after ESAL with subcutaneous hematomas probably due to early drainage removing.

4. Discussion

Al-Marhoon MS et al. performed an open cystolithotomy, endourological transurethral, and percuteneous litholapaxy of vesicle stones in children. They concluded that an open and endourological management of vesical stones in children is efficient, with low incidence of complications, but an open cystolithotomy seems to be safer (Al-Marhoon et al., 2009). Wollin TA et al. performed a percutaneous suprapubic cystolithotomy in cases of bladder stones larger than 3 cm or multiple stones with 1 cm size. They used nephroscope and pneumatic lithotripter (Wollin et al., 1999).

Miller DC et Park JM described a percutaneous approach for treatment of the stone in an augmented bladder. They inserted a laparoscopic trocar and via endobag extracted the stone without lithotripsy (Miller & Park , 2003). Segarra J. et al. inserting a Hasson trocar through the 1.5 cm suprapubic incision were able via the trocar to disintegrate and extract the stone fragments (Segarra et al., 2001). Some authors report laparoscopic resection in rear cases of urachal cyst containing stones employ a laparoscopic transabdominal approach with or without bladder wall resection (Ansari & Hemal, 2002; Okegawa, 2006; Pust, 2007; Yohannes 2003). Colegate-Stone TJ et al. reported a case of bladder wall injury and bladder stone formation after inguinal herniorrhaphy, treated laparoscopicaly (Colegate-Stone et al., 2008). Ingber MS et al. reported a novel technique for removal of intravesical polypropylene mesh through a single laparoscopic port directly from the bladder (Ingber MS et al.,2009). Reddy BS and Daniel RD described a new technique for extraction of complex foreign bodies from the urinary bladder using cystoscopy while the bladder remains insufflated with carbon dioxide (Reddy & Daniel, 2004). Eradi B and Shenoy MU. describing the similar procedures and named it laparoscopic. Actually they used a laparoscopic trocar, but not the laparoscopic method (Eradi & Shenoy, 2008).

Author	Operative Technique	Indications	Number of cases
Al-Marhoon MS et al 2009	open cystolithotomy, endourological transurethral, and percuteneous litholapaxy	vesicle stones in children	107 Open – 53 Endoscopic – 54 (23 transurethral and 24 suprapubic)
Wollin et al., 1999	percutaneous suprapubic cystolithotomy with nephroscope and pneumatic lithotripter	bladder stones larger than 3 cm or multiple stones with 1 cm size	15
Miller & Park , 2003	percutaneous approach in augmented bladder with laparoscopic trocar and via endobag. Extraction of the stones without lithotripsy.	treatment of the stones in augmented urinary bladder	4 (one case conversion)
Segarra et al., 2001	Disintegrating and extracting the fragments from the stones via the Hasson trocar through the 1.5 cm suprapubic incision	stones in urinary bladder	20
Ansari & Hemal, 2002; Okegawa, 2006; Pust, 2007	laparoscopic resection of urachal cyst	urachal cyst containing stones	6
Yohannes P et al. 2003	laparoscopic resection of urachal cyst	urachal cyst without stones	1
Colegate-Stone et al., 2008	Laparoscopy extraction from urinary bladder	bladder stone formation after inguinal herniorrhaphy	1
Reddy & Daniel, 2004	cystoscopy and optical device through the urethra, a 10-mm laparoscopic port introduced suprapubically for extraction of complex foreign bodies	foreign bodies in urinary bladder	1
Ingber MS et al. 2009	Single port suprapubic extraction of foreign bodies in urinary bladder	foreign bodies in urinary bladder	2

Table 1. Data showing operative techniques, indications and number of cases for treatment of urinary bladder stones from different authors

5. Conclusion

There are two main methods for surgical treatment of urinary bladder stones - open suprapubic cystolithotomy and transurethral lithotripsy with litholapaxy. These two methods are combined by many authors, others perform endoscopic techniques using laparoscopic instruments or laparoscopy as operative method. Our endoscopic method is based on the principles of the open cystolithotomy, but completely laparoendoscopic extraperitonealy. Because of this we named our technique Endoscopic Sectio Alta. To the best of our knowledge this is the first application of such a technique.

In conclusion, Endoscopic Sectio Alta for urinary bladder stones treatment is simple and safe laparoscopic technique, which has not been described untill now. The procedure avoids urethral damage and prevents the patient from open procedures. In selected cases of men without residual urine, who do not want prostate surgery, our technique is the treatment method of choice, especially in a laparoscopic clinic. In addition, this simple technique may be very useful as a training procedure in laparoscopy. Further cases are necessary for better results and indications.

6. Acknowledgement

This work has been supported by the Bulgarian ministry of education, youth and science under grant number DDVU-02-105/2010.

7. References

Al-Marhoon MS, Sarhan OM, Awad BA et al. 2009. Comparison of endourological and open cystolithotomy in the management of bladder stones in children. *J Urol.* Jun;181(6):2684-7;

Ansari MS, Hemal AK. 2002. A rare case of urachovesical calculus: a diagnostic dilemma and endo-laparoscopic management. *J Laparoendosc Adv Surg Tech A.* Aug;12(4):281-3.

Chow KS, Chou CY. 2008. A boy with a large bladder stone. *Pediatr Neonatol.* Aug;49(4):150-3

Colegate-Stone TJ, Raymond T, Khot U et al. 2008. Laparoscopic management of iatrogenic bladder injury and bladder stone formation following laparoscopic inguinal herniorrhaphy. *Hernia.* Aug;12(4):429-30.

Eradi B, Shenoy MU. 2008. Laparoscopic extraction of the awkward intravesical foreign body: a point of technique. *Surg Laparosc Endosc Percutan Tech.* Feb;18(1):75-6.

H Ellis. A history of bladder stone. 1979. *J R Soc Med.* April; 72(4): 248–25

Holman E, Khan AM, Flasko T et al. 2004. Endoscopic management of pediatric urolithiasis in a developing country.*Urology.* Jan;63(1):159-62.

Ingber MS, Stein RJ, Rackley RR et al. 2009. Single-port Transvesical Excision of Foreign Body in the Bladder. *Urology.* Dec;74(6):1347-50.

Miller DC, Park JM. 2003. Percutaneous cystolithotomy using a laparoscopic entrapment sac. *Urology.* Aug;62(2):333-6.

Okegawa T, Odagane A, Nutahara K et al. 2006. Laparoscopic management of urachal remnants in adulthood. *Int J Urol.*;13:1466–1469.

Pust A, Ovenbeck R, Erbersdobler A et al. 2007. Laparoscopic management of patent urachus in an adult man.*Urol Int.*;79(2):184-6.

Reddy BS, Daniel RD. 2004. A novel laparoscopic technique for removal of foreign bodies from the urinary bladder using carbon dioxide insufflation. *Surg Laparosc Endosc Percutan Tech.* Aug;14(4):238-9.

Segarra J, Palou J, Montlleó M et al. 2001. Hasson's laparoscopic trocar in percutaneous bladder stone lithotripsy. *Int Urol Nephrol.*;33(4):625-6.

Seo IY, Han DY, Oh SJ et al. 2008. Laparoscopic excision of a urachal cyst containing large stones in an adult. Yonsei Med J. Oct 31;49(5):869-71.

Schwartz BF, Stoller ML. 2000. The vesical calculus. *Urol Clin North Am.* May;27(2):333-46.

Stolzenburg JU, Do M, Pfeiffer H et al. 2002. The endoscopic extraperitoneal radical prostatectomy (EERPE): technique and initial experience. World J Urol. May;20(1):48-55.

Tugcu V, Polat H, Ozbay B et al. 2009. Percutaneous versus transurethral cystolithotripsy. *J Endourol.* Feb;23(2):237-41.

Wollin TA, Singal RK, Whelan T et al. 1999. Percutaneous suprapubic cystolithotripsy for treatment of large bladder calculi. *J Endourol.* Dec;13(10):739-44.

Yohannes P, Bruno T, Pathan M et al. 2003. Laparoscopic radical excision of urachal sinus. *J Endourol.* Sep;17(7):475-9.

7

Laparoscopy Training Courses in Urology

Sutchin R Patel and Stephen Y Nakada
Department of Urology,
University of Wisconsin School of Medicine and Public Health
United States

1. Introduction

The history of laparoscopic surgery began with man's attempts to inspect concealed areas of the body. Early endoscopy from Bozzini's "lichtleiter" in 1805 to the development of modern cystoscopy by Nitze in the late 1800s helped develop the optical tools required for laparoscopy. The early 1900s saw the birth of laparoscopy with Kelling, a surgeon from Dresden, describing the technique of celioscopy in dogs and Jacobaeus from Sweden reporting two cases of thoraco-laparoscopy in which he used a trocar to create pneumoperitoneum in humans and then inserted a cystoscope. Kurt Semm, an engineer and gynecologist helped develop many of the other tools associated with laparoscopy including an automatic insufflation device that monitored gas flow and intra-abdominal pressure, thermocoagulation for use during the procedure as well as many early laparoscopy instruments. (Gomella & Strup, 1994)

The first laparoscopic nephrectomy was performed by Clayman and colleagues in 1990. (Clayman et al., 1991) With improvements and refinement of the technology, the first laparoscopic living donor nephrectomy soon followed. (Ratner et al., 1995) In 1997, Nakada and colleagues, performed the first hand-assisted laparoscopic nephrectomy (HALN) with a sleeve in the United States. (Nakada et al., 1997) By placing a hand in the abdomen, the HALN provided urologists tactile sensation and helped decrease the learning curve for laparoscopy. (Gaston KE et al., 2004) The hand-assisted approach also allowed older urologists that had not been trained in laparoscopy to begin to perform laparoscopic cases and helped bridge the gap from open surgery and a pure laparoscopic approach. (Munver R et al., 2004)

With the rapid advances in technology in the field of urology, post-graduate training courses are important to help bridge the technology gap for current practicing urologists. The development of newer high-fidelity simulators and metrics for assessing laparoscopic skill acquisition are essential in order for us to better teach laparoscopic surgery.

2. The learning curve for laparoscopy

The application of any new technology is associated with a learning curve. In laparoscopy, the ability to translate a 2-dimensional perspective on the monitor into 3-dimensional movements inside the body, the loss of tactile sensation, the limitations of using fixed port sites which limit mobility (limited degrees of freedom: yaw, pitch, roll, insertion plus actuation of the instrument) and the fulcrum effect make the transition from open surgery to laparoscopy challenging. (Kumar & Gill, 2006) Despite these shortcomings, some of the limitations can be overcome with compensatory mechanisms such as motion parallax to estimate depth and frequently touching objects in the visual field to obtain some tactile input.

Figert et al. found that a specific set of laparoscopic skills may not aid the transfer of training to a different set of laparoscopic skills and that open surgical experience does not improve the transfer of training to acquiring new laparoscopic skills. (Figert et al, 2001) They concluded that specific minimally invasive training is needed to develop laparoscopic surgery skills.

There is evidence to suggest that intensive training in the setting of a formal fellowship decreases the learning curve for laparoscopy. Cadeddu and colleagues identified no difference in the complication rates between the initial 20 to 40 laparoscopic cases compared to subsequent cases for 13 surgeons that had completed at least 1 year of fellowship training in laparoscopic surgery. (Cadeddu et al., 2001) The authors also found no change in the open conversion rate with time and concluded that the experience acquired during intensive laparoscopic training may decrease the learning curve needed to achieve proficiency.

Though the learning curve for laparoscopic surgery remains less well defined and may be different for individual surgeons and different procedures, a number of different studies have tried to estimate the learning curve for laparoscopic radical nephrectomy, donor nephrectomy and prostatectomy. (Table 1.) Phillips et al. studied a single center's learning curve for laparoscopic retroperitoneal radical nephrectomy. (Phillips et al., 2005) There was a significant difference in the operative time for the last 30 cases compared to all cases in the series. There was no significant difference between blood loss, conversion rate or complication rate between the last 30 cases compared to all cases. The authors did show a decrease in conversion to open surgery from 4 cases to 2 cases when comparing cases 1-20 to cases 21-40 but did not comment on how many cases constituted the learning curve for the procedure. Jeon et al. evaluated the outcomes for three novice surgeons and their first 50 laparoscopic radical nephrectomies. (Jeon et al., 2009) The authors found a significant difference in the estimated blood loss (236 vs 191cc, $p=0.04$) and transfusion rate (17.8% vs 4.8%, $p=0.02$) when comparing each surgeons' first 15 cases compared to their remaining 35 cases. There was a significant difference in operating time between the first 15 cases in the series compared to the last 15 cases but no significant difference in intraoperative complications or conversions to open surgery. The authors concluded that 15 cases were required for a novice surgeon to achieve competence in laparoscopic radical nephrectomy.

The laparoscopic approach for partial nephrectomy can be a challenging procedure requiring a surgeon to be experienced in general laparoscopic renal surgery as well as be facile with intracorporeal suturing in order to achieve hemostasis and reconstruction of the kidney within a reasonable warm ischemia time. Link et al. investigated a single institutional learning curve for laparoscopic partial nephrectomy. (Link et al., 2005) Linear regression analysis revealed that total operative time decreased significantly with increasing surgeon experience. Warm ischemia time increased significantly with larger tumor diameter but was not related to surgeon experience.

Hruza et al. evaluated the learning curve for three generations of surgeons that performed 2200 laparoscopic radical prostatectomies. (Hruza et al., 2010) First generation surgeons were defined as surgeons with a great deal of experience in open surgery but no laparoscopic training. Second generation surgeons were surgeons with open surgery

Procedure-Study	No. Cases (No. Surgeons)	Learning Curve Parameter(s) Studied	Results
LRN-Phillips et al., 2005	121 (NR)	OR Time, Conversion Rate, Intraop Complications	OR Time: All Cases=140 min; Last 30 Cases=120 min (p=0.012) Conversion: N=7 in first 60 cases (none after that) Intraop Complications: N=9 in first 60 cases; N=3 in last 61 cases
LRN-Jeon et al., 2009	150 (3)	OR Time, Conversion Rate, Intraop Complications	Mean OR Time: 188 min (statistically significant difference in OR time between first 15 cases and last 15 cases); Conversion: N=1(2.2%) in first 45 cases; N=2 (1.9%)in remaining 105 Cases Intraop Complications N=6 (13.3%) in first 45 cases; N=9(8.6%) in remaining 105 cases
LPN-Link et al., 2005	178 (1)	OR Time, Warm Ischemia Time	Statistically significant decrease in OR time with increasing surgeon experience. (p=0.003) Warm ischemia time is related to resected tumor size (p=0.005) but not to surgeon experience (p=0.96).
LRP-Hruza et al., 2010	2200 (5 surgeons performed 96% of cases)	Complication Free Rate	Overall Complication Free Rate: 1st Gen (Cases 1-50)=54% 2nd Gen(Cases 1-50)=60% 3rd Gen (Cases 1-50)=61% 1st Gen (Cases 201-250)=62% 2nd Gen(Cases 151-200)=58% 3rd Gen (Cases 201-250)=75%
LRP-Secin et al., 2010	8544 (51)	Positive Surgical Margin Rate	Positive Surgical Margin Rate: 22% Absolute risk difference for 10 vs 250 prior surgeries=4.8%

Table 1. Assessment of Learning Curves for Urologic Procedures. LRN: Laparoscopic Radical Nephrectomy; LPN: Laparoscopic Partial Nephrectomy; LRP: Laparoscopic Radical Prostatectomy; NR: Not Reported; OR: Operating Room; Intraop: Intraoperative; Gen: Generation

experience that were trained by the first generation surgeons in laparoscopy and third generation surgeons had no or limited open surgery training that were trained by both the first and second generation surgeons in laparoscopy. Though the technique for laparoscopic radical prostatectomy was not constant (first 871 patients: transperitoneal; remaining 1329 patients retroperitoneal) over the time of the study (1999-2008), the authors showed a higher complication-free rate for third generation surgeons in their first 50 cases and their last 50 cases (cases 201-250) when compared to first generation surgeons. The authors conclude that the individual learning curve for third generation surgeons was shorter when compared to first and second generation surgeons and this may be due to their dedicated learning program. In an international multicenter study, Secin et al. studied the learning curve for laparoscopic radical prostatectomy performed on 8,544 consecutive patients by 51 surgeons from 14 academic institutions in Europe and the United States. (Secin et al., 2010) The authors investigated the learning curve of laparoscopic radical prostatectomy for positive surgical margins and compared it to a published learning curve for open radical prostatectomy. There was an improvement in surgical margin rates up to a plateau at 200 to 250 surgeries with an absolute risk difference for 10 vs 250 prior surgeries of 4.8% (95% CI 1.5,8.5). Neither surgeon generation nor prior open radical prostatectomy experience improved the margin rate suggesting that the positive surgical margin rate is primarily a function of laparoscopic training and experience.

The learning curve for procedures can be difficult to compare even between studies on the same procedure since results (such as operative time, conversions, intraoperative complications, blood loss or positive margin status) are not always reported and when they are reported they are not reported in quartiles or in terms of which case they occurred in the series. It is also important to realize that the learning curve for a procedure may differ for each individual surgeon. Given that many of the papers in the literature are carried out at large academic institutions, the learning curve for surgeons in community practice with limited case access may be different.

For urologists that were not trained in laparoscopy, hand-assisted laparoscopic surgery can serve as a bridge between open surgery and laparoscopy. The loss of tactile sensation is one major factor that prolongs the learning curve for laparoscopic surgery. Having a hand in the abdomen can help provide tactile sensation as well as allow an easier method to retract tissue and aid in dissection. Hand-assisted surgery thus makes it easier and safer to transition from open surgery to laparoscopy for surgeons that have not received formal training in laparoscopy. Gaston et al. demonstrated a short learning curve for hand-assisted laparoscopic radical nephrectomy via decreasing difficulty scores and operative times in as few as 4 cases. (Gaston et al., 2004) The oncologic, operative and postoperative results for hand-assisted laparoscopic radical nephrectomy have been shown to be comparable to standard laparoscopy and thus may be an advantageous approach early in a surgeon's experience or for cases involving larger tumors. (Nelson et al., 2002)

3. Laparoscopic training courses

With the increased prevalence of laparoscopy in urology, reliable training and assessment of skill become increasingly important. Laparoscopic skills are not an innate behavior, nor can they be easily learned by observation or through reading surgical texts and can only be acquired through hands-on training. (Emken et al., 2004) Because of the unique nature of the laparoscopic skill set, teaching these skills requires an increased emphasis on practical and skills training. (Derossis et al., 1998; Scott et al., 2001) Laparoscopy is different from open surgery in that its performed using long instruments inserted through ports made in the skin. The laparoscopic instruments can amplify tremor and because of the fulcrum effect movement of the instruments outside of the body correspond to movement in the opposite direction inside the body. Furthermore laparoscopy requires ambidexterity, manipulation from a 2-dimensional magnified image on the monitor to 3-dimensional movement inside the abdomen and working with minimal tactile feedback.

A number of post-graduate laparoscopy courses are available for urologists that did not receive this type of training in residency. Because of the rapidly evolving technology in the field of urology, post-graduate courses are important to allow the practicing urologist to stay current by learning new surgical techniques. The post-graduate courses come in one to two day sessions or longer "mini-fellowships" (5-day course) and usually involve didactic sessions, animal or cadaver laboratories, inanimate model training and case observation or videos. (Table 2.)

Study	Survey Resp/Tot (% RR)	Course Description	Course Components	Follow-Up	Results
Kolla et al., 2010	1 yr: 77% 2 yr: 65% 3 yr: 68% (Tot=106)	5-day laparoscopic ablative or laparoscopic reconstructive renal surgery mini-fellowship	• Tutorial sessions with mentors • Inanimate model skills training • Animal laboratory skills training • OR observation	Range: 1 to 3 years post-course	• 5-day mini-fellowship successfully increases case volume and advances the complexity of laparoscopic procedures they perform in practice up to 3 years after the course
Pareek et al., 2008	32/52 (61%)	2-day AUA Mentored Laparoscopy course (2002-2003)	• Didactic and video presentations • Inanimate model skills training • Animal model skills training • Videotape mentoring	Mean: 48 months (Range:41 to 55 months)	• 97% of respondents stated that their laparoscopic practice had expanded since taking the course • 81% stated that video mentoring was helpful in laparoscopic skills acquisition
Marguet et al., 2004	56/71 (79%)	1-day hand-assisted laparoscopy post-graduate training course	• Didactic • Technique Instruction • Animal laboratory	Range: 6 months to 1 year post-course	• Respondents who completed course and underwent mentoring by course instructor or another experienced laparoscopist were more likely (93%) to perform lap cases than those who were not mentored (44%) ($p<0.001$)

Study	Survey Resp/Tot (% RR)	Course Description	Course Components	Follow-Up	Results
Colegrove et al., 1999	168/322 (52%)	2-day university sponsored post-graduate laparoscopic training course	• Didactic • Live video presentations • ▪ Animal model skills training • ▪ Laparoscopy simulator laboratory	Range: 4.5 to 7 years post-course	• 54% had performed 1 or more lap procedures in past year (>4.5 yr after course) compared to 84% 1 yr after taking the course

Table 2. Description of Laparoscopy Training Courses and Results of Follow-Up Surveys. Survey Resp/Tot: Number of survey respondents/Total number of urologists taking the course; RR: survey response rate (%); lap:laparoscopy; yr: year

Rane describes a 9-phase mini-fellowship training model for urologic laparoscopic surgery. (RaneA, 2005) Phase 1 is completion of a basic and advanced training course and an animal laboratory prior to the mini-fellowship. Phase 2 is practice at home or in the office using pelvic trainers with phase 3 proceeding to an animal laboratory course. Phase 4 incorporates visits to centers of international repute to observe high-volume laparoscopic urology followed by observing the mentor perform several major renal laparoscopic cases in phase 5. the trainee then performs several hand-assisted renal procedures under direct mentor guidance at the mentor hospital in phase 6 with the trainee then advancing to perform laparoscopic or retroperitoneoscopic renal surgeries in phase 7 under the mentor's guidance. In phase 8 the trainee mentors and assists other trainees to start laparoscopic surgery at their own hospitals prior to practicing laparoscopy independently in the final phase. Though this is a very thorough and comprehensive fellowship model and it is reported that 9 trainees have participated in the fellowship over 36 months it is unclear how much time the fellowship takes or if there is any objective data on follow-up or incorporation of laparoscopic skills into their practice.

Pansodoro et al describe a 4 step program consisting of observation, theoretical learning, assisting and operating to teach laparoscopy. Fourteen trainees underwent this training program from 2001 to 2005. One year after completing the program, 12 out of the 14 trainees were performing laparoscopic urology at their home institution. They reported no major complications and their conversion rate was <2%.

3.1 Surgical mentoring

Mentoring surgeons early in their laparoscopic experience has been shown to shorten the learning curve and lower the complication rates. (Fabrizio et al., 2003) Video mentoring allows an instructor to better critique laparoscopic performance and technique in order to help a course participant better improve the basic skills required for laparoscopy. (Hedican & Nakada, 2007) Nakada et al showed that expert videotape mentoring and analysis of laparoscopic skills training of urologists during an AUA-sponsored hands-on laparoscopy course can improve laparoscopic skills gained during the course. (Nakada et al., 2004) In a survey of participants of a mentored laparoscopy course, Pareek et al found that 81% of course respondents felt that videotape mentoring was valuable. (Pareek et al., 2008)

Marguet et al. showed that mentoring post-graduate urologists for their initial hand-assisted laparoscopic case after taking a hand-assisted laparoscopy course lead to greater integration of laparoscopy into a community based urology practice. (Marguet et al., 2004) A survey was sent to 71 urologists who had taken the hand-assisted laparoscopy course with 53% of the course participants receiving post-course mentoring. Ninety three percent of the mentored surgeons trained in hand-assisted laparoscopy were performing these operations compared to only 44% of the non-mentored participants 6 months after the course. Shalhav and colleagues further incorporated the mentoring relationship into their training method. (Shalhav et al., 2002) Participants completed a standard animate and inanimate training course and then entered into mentorship training with their instructor. The training included an observational period where the participant watched a number of procedures at their mentor's hospital followed by the instructor then assisting the trainee in complex laparoscopic operations at the trainee's hospital. Of the two surgeons trained via this method, one performed 30 laparoscopic cases in the first 8 months and the other 10 cases in the first 3 months after completion of the course. Fabrizio et al have also reported that expert mentoring can also be valuable to experienced laparoscopists learning a new complex procedure such as laparoscopic radical prostatectomy. (Fabrizio et al.,2003) Despite the benefits of more rapid skills acquisition from mentorship following completion of a laparoscopic training course, the time commitment required by both the trainee and mentoring surgeon and the need to obtain temporary operating privileges and malpractice coverage at another hospital can both be a significant obstacles to overcome. (Hedican & Nakada, 2007)

4. Competency in laparoscopy

Reports revealing the prevalence of medical errors has prompted calls for closer scrutiny of surgical training and practice. (Hasson HM, 2006; Cushieri A, 1995) The Accreditation Council of Graduate Medical Education (ACGME) has identified six core competencies (patient care, medical knowledge, professionalism, system-based practice, practice-based learning and interpersonal/communication skills) to define competence. (Kavic MS, 2002) These 6 competencies are pertinent to laparoscopic surgeons in their ability to care for their patients. The competencies of patient care and medical knowledge encompass the cognitive and technical skills that are unique to laparoscopy and include: 1.) pre-operative care: diagnosis, pre-operative preparation and medical judgement 2.) operative performance: cognitive and technical skills, intra-operative judgement 3.) post-operative care: monitoring, treatment and medical judgement. (Hasson HM, 2006)

Assessing cognitive skills in laparoscopy requires that the surgeon be able to correctly diagnose the situation, assess patients that would be adequate candidates for laparoscopic surgery, understand the physiology of pneumoperitoneum and entry, be able to diagnose and manage intra-operative and post-operative complications and manage the patient post-operatively. These skills are generally taught via didactic lectures and operative videos and tested with multiple-choice tests or discussion of patient management scenarios. Almost all of the post-graduate laparoscopy courses have some didactic or lecture component to address cognitive skills.

The technical skills required to perform laparoscopic surgery can be more difficult to assess. The skills a surgeon needs to acquire include the ability to operate in a 3-dimensional field using the 2-dimensional image on a video screen, adapt to the restricted space/freedom in the abdomen, be comfortable with the limited instrument manipulations due to the fulcrum effect and minimal tactile feedback. Laparoscopic training courses focus on helping a trainee develop these skills via both inanimate skills training as well as via an animal laboratory. Newly developed computer-based simulators constitute a new paradigm in laparoscopic surgery training which allow for more objective measurement of laparoscopic skills.

5. Surgical simulation

A simulator is defined as "a device that enables the operator to reproduce or represent under test conditions phenomena likely to occur in actual performance" and thus a surgical simulator describes any model used to represent surgery (from box trainers to cadaveric models to virtual reality models). (Wignall et al., 2008) The different types of simulation can be categorized by the concept of fidelity. Low fidelity simulators such as box trainers are those that do not accurately mimic the surgical environment. Despite the lack of realism in these simulators, low fidelity simulators can be important in teaching basic surgical techniques such as laparoscopic knot tying and tend to be low cost and generally portable. High fidelity simulators are those that are more lifelike and can be used to teach an entire operation. These include animal or cadaveric models as well as newly developed virtual reality simulators.

5.1 Simulator validation

In order for a simulator to be used to assess competence, it must be evaluated objectively to determine its reliability and validity. (McDougall EM, 2007) The reliability of a training instrument refers to the reproducibility of the test. A given simulator must be consistent in its subject measurement not just with a single trainee on different occasions but also among different trainees. Validity implies that an instrument appropriately measures what it was intended to measure. Face validity establishes that a test seems reasonable and appropriate and is usually assessed by nonexperts in relation to its realism. Content validity assures that the contents of the test cover the relevant areas of the subject being assessed. Face and content validity are relatively subjective appraisals and objective validity assessments (criterion validity, construct validity) are more challenging and time consuming. Criterion validity correlates the results of a new assessment tool with those of an established tool. Criterion validity is composed of concurrent validity (the extent to which a simulator correlates with the "gold standard") and predictive validity (a measure of if a simulator predicts future performance). Construct validity is established by demonstrating differences in test performance between experts and novices in the measured skill and is considered one of the most valuable assessments of a simulator before it is accepted as a competency-evaluating device. (McDougall EM, 2007) In order to validate a simulator the simulator must accurately predict performance in the operating room, however, because there are few reliable measures of surgical performance this can be difficult to achieve. (Wignall et al., 2008)

5.2 Pelvic trainer

The pelvic trainer is one of the simplest methods to acquire preliminary laparoscopic skill. It is easy to use and allows surgeons to gain synchronization of both hands in completing a task. The pelvic trainer allows the surgeon to get acclimated to working in a 3-dimensional space based on a 2-dimensional view and is useful in allowing the surgeon to gain experience in knot tying. Several low-cost pelvic trainers (camera-less, mirrored box trainers) are available, they may be useful for simple laparoscopic skills but the absence of a camera may also further decrease the fidelity of the simulator as it would not mimic the external set-up and optics during laparoscopy. (Rassweiler et al., 2007) A number of "homemade recipes" for creating laparoscopic box trainers are available in the literature. Though these are relatively low fidelity trainers, they may be helpful in practicing basic laparoscopic skills (object transfer, cutting, suturing, knot tying). (Chung et al., 2005; Blacker AJR, 2005) Construct validity of pelvic box trainers has been shown by Katz et al, who compared the performance of 44 urologists with different levels of laparoscopic experience (beginners, basic, advanced). A significant difference was found among all of the groups (sensitivity: 71-85%, specificity of 74-88%) A modification of a closed mechanical simulator is the P.O.P trainer which provides pulsating organ perfusion. (Szinicz et al., 2001) The central artery of porcine organs or organ complexes (aorta) is catheterized and connected to a pump on the trainer. The perfusion medium (red colored tap water) is delivered into the organ by the pump. This system can thus allow a higher fidelity simulator and allow one to practice surgical procedures (nephrectomy, partial nephrectomy, retroperitoneal lymph node dissection) and allow for the management of arterial bleeding. However the cost of the simulator is considerable and literature on validation is still lacking. (Autorino et al., 2010)

Low Fidelity [a]
- Mirrored box trainer (no camera)
- Box trainer with camera
- Hybrid trainer (similar to box trainer containing organ/tissue)
- Perfused Organ Pelvic trainer (POP Trainer)

High Fidelity (Biological)
- Animal Models (Porcine)
- Human Cadaver Model

High Fidelity (Virtual Reality)
- MIST-VR
- LapSim Laparoscopic Trainer (Surgical Science Ltd, Sweden)

Table 3. Types of Simulators for Laparoscopic Surgery in Urology. a: increasing fidelity in descending order from mirrored box trainer to POP trainer

5.3 Animal and cadaveric models

Once a trainee has acquired skill working in inanimate models, an animal model is the next step and will allow the surgeon to work in an environment similar to humans. The porcine model is one of the most commonly used animal models and the trainee can gain confidence in obtaining access and pneumoperitoneum and trocar positioning as well as performing the laparoscopic surgical procedure of choice. The animal model allows the surgeon to use all of the same instruments (bipolar or monopolar cautery, clips, stapling devices, hemostatic agents) that he or she would use during laparoscopic surgery as well as allow for similar risk of complications (vascular injury, bowel injury, splenic or liver injury) without harming a human patient.

Cadaveric models have also been used to teach laparoscopy. Cadavers offer the advantage of helping the trainee gain a perspective of real macroscopic anatomy of all of the organs and structures. Thus spatial perception of anatomy is improved in this model and allows the surgeon to better understand laparoscopic landmarks. (Katz et al., 2003) However, cadaver models do have a number of disadvantages: 1) they do not bleed and thus no hemostasis is required 2) endoscopic vision during the case is always clear 3) tissues dissection is not comparable to a live human being 4) work on cadavers is potentially dangerous due to the risk of the transmission of hematogenous diseases 5) like the porcine model, the cadaveric model can also be expensive. (Piechaud PT & Pansadoro A, 2006)

5.4 Virtual reality simulation

Virtual reality is a new category of simulation that has arisen due to the technologic advances in graphics and computing. Virtual reality is defined as "an artificial environment which is experienced through sensory stimuli provided by a computer and in which one's actions partially determine what happens in the environment." (Wignall et al., 2008) Though virtual reality simulators are fairly expensive and require maintenance, they offer the opportunity to practice basic skills or entire surgical operations in a virtual environment. For a virtual reality simulator to be realistic and valuable it must correctly reproduce anatomy, preserve anatomical characteristics such as weight and deformability and ideally provide some form of tactile feedback. These characteristics can allow for the simulation of mistakes in the virtual environment such as bleeding or injury to other adjacent organs and thus more realistically provide feedback to the surgeon.

Virtual reality simulators can also enhance the evaluation of a trainee by measuring task performance. The Minimally Invasive Surgical Trainer-Virtual Reality (MIST-VR) was one of the first simulators to automatically record a number of different objective measures such as number of errors, time taken for task completion and economy of path length. (Undre & Darzi, 2007) The MIST-VR set-up includes a frame with 2 laparoscopic instruments attached to it linked to a computer. The system also allows one to train on simple tasks such as picking and placing objects and suturing prior to performing complete procedures. The MIST trainer was able to distinguish between grades of surgeons (construct validity) and was shown to predict performance in the operating room (predictive validity). (Taffinder et al., 1998; Maithel et al., 2005; Seymour et al., 2002) Seymour et al performed a prospective, randomized, double-blinded study that demonstarated that virtual reality training transfers technical skills to the operating.

The LapSim virtual reality trainer (Surgical Science Ltd.) developed in Sweden is a personal computer-based system with a monitor and a laparoscopic interface set-up that includes 2 instruments and a foot pedal. The software for the system consists of a number of modules that can train a surgeon in basic laparoscopic skills (camera navigation, instrument manipulation: grasping, cutting, clipping, suturing). Construct validity has been demonstrated in several studies for the LapSim trainer. (Duffy et al., 2005; Ericksen et al., 2005) Currently the surgery modules for the LapSim trainer include cholecystectomy, appendectomy and gynecologic module (tubal occlusion, salpingectomy, myoma suturing) but no urologic procedure modules have been developed to date.

6. Laparoscopic skills assessment and course follow-up

Despite the literature on laparoscopic training courses and various laparoscopic simulators, more studies need to be performed that objectively measure laparoscopic skill acquisition along with long-term follow-up of course participants. Criteria used to demonstrate competency in the past have included the number of procedures performed, time taken to complete a case or evaluation by senior surgeons. (Dent TL, 1991; European Association of Endoscopic Surgeons, 1994) However, these criteria are known to be crude and indirect measures of technical skill or to suffer from the influence of subjectivity or bias. (Aggarwal et al., 2004) With the increasing need to assess surgical performance objectively, dexterity analysis and video-based assessment have begun to be used.

The movement of laparoscopic instruments and the surgeon's hands have both been used to help assess surgical performance. Smith et al connected laparoscopic forceps to sensors to map their position in space and relay the movements to a personal computer. This allowed for calculation fo the instrument's total path length which was then compared to the minimum path length required to complete a task. (Smith et al., 2001) The Imperial College Surgical Assessment Device (ICSAD) has sensors placed on the back of a surgeon's hands and studies have confirmed construct validity of the ICSAD as a surgical assessment device for both simple tasks and for surgical procedures. (Taffinder et al., 1999; Torkington et al., 2001; Smith et al., 2002) Experienced laparoscopic surgeons made significantly fewer movements than occasional laparoscopists who were better than novices in the field. The ICSAD device has also been shown to objectively assess the acquisition of psychomotor skill of trainees attending laparoscopic training courses. (Aggarwal et al., 2004)

Martin et al developed a video-based assessment of operative skill, the Objective Structured Assessment of Technical Skill (OSATS). (Martin et al., 1997) OSATS involves 6 tasks on a bench format with direct observation and assesment on a task-specific checklist, a seven-item global rating sore and a pass/fail evaluation. Twenty surgeons in training of differing experience level performed equivalent open surgical tasks on the bench format and then on live anesthetized animals. There was excellent correlation between assessment on the bench and live models. Test/retest and inter-rater reliabilities were higher for global scores, making them a more reliable and valid measurement tool. OSATS can be used to help assess concurrent validity if a simulator performance score correlates with the OSATS performance score on an accepted evaluating model. OSATS can thus also be used to assess predictive validity. (McDougall EM, 2007) It should be noted that the OSATS performance score evaluation is time consuming as the assessment of 20 surgical trainees on the OSATS required 48 examiners for 3 hours each. (Martin et al., 1997) To achieve instant and more objective feedback on a surgeon's technical skills, virtual reality simulation may be more useful. Studies to confirm the role of virtual reality simulators as assessment devices have concentrated on the demonstration of construct validity, with experienced surgeons completing the tasks on the MIST-VR significantly faster, with lower rates of error and greater economy of movement scores. (Gallagher et al., 2001)

When assessing the impact of laparoscopy training courses, there is limited long-term data on the incorporation of laparoscopy into clinical practice. Of urologists that had participated in laparoscopic training courses at the University of Iowa in 1991, 84% of respondents had performed at least 1 laparoscopic case at 1 year follow-up. (See et al., 1994) However, 5 year follow-up for the same group of urologists revealed a decline to 54%. (Colegrove et al., 1999) Pareek et al surveyed urologists taking a mentored laparoscopy course in 2002 and 2003 with a mean follow-up of 48 months found that 97% of respondents stated that their laparoscopic practice had expanded. (Pareek et al., 2008) Kolla et al surveyed urologists that had completed their 5-day mini-fellowhip in laparoscopic surgery found that 72%, 71% and 71% of respondents performed laparoscopic renal surgery at 1,2 and 3 years respectively since completing the course. (Kolla et al., 2010) Though it appears that there is good incorporation of laparoscopic surgery into clinical practice, more studies with long-term (> 5 years) follow-up are required to better assess the impact of post-graduate courses.

7. Conclusions

The exponential rise and incorporation of technology in urology has fueled the need for better post-graduate laparoscopic courses and methods to aid urologists in skill acquisition. Training courses have been shown to help decrease the learning curve associated with laparoscopy and the need has diminished as more and more trainees are fully trained in the technique. More studies with long term follow-up are needed to better assess incorporation of laparoscopy into urologists' clinical practice. Though a number of different simulators are available to help with laparoscopic skill acquisition and even for certification purposes, it is important that simulators undergo thorough validation testing prior to being approved for competency assessment.

8. References

Aggarwal R, Moorthy K, Darzi A. (2004). Laparoscopic skills training assesment. *British Journal of Surgery*, Vol.91, No.12, pp. 1549-1558, ISSN 1365-2168

Aggarwal R, Hance J, Moorthy K, Munz Y, Undre S, Darzi A. (2004). Assessment of psychomotor skills acquisition during laparoscopic cholecystectomy courses. *American Journal of Surgery*, Vol.190, No.3, pp. 507-511, ISSN 1879-1883

Bergman S, Feldman LS, Anidjar M, Demyttenaere SV, Carli F, Metrakos P, Tchervenkov J, Paraskevas S, Fried GM. (2008). "First, do no harm": monitoring outcomes during the transition from open to laparoscopic live donor nephrectomy in a Canadian centre. *Canadian Journal of Surgery*, Vol.51, No.2, pp. 103-110, ISSN 1488-2310

Blacker AJ. (2005). How to build your own laparoscopic trainer. *Journal of Endourology*, Vol.19, No.6, pp. 748-752, ISSN 1557-900X

Caddedu JA, Wolf JS Jr, Nakada SY, Chen R, Shalhav A, Bishoff JT, Hamilton B, Schulam PG, Dunn M, Hoenig D, Fabrizio M, Hedican S, Averch TD. (2001). Complications of laparoscopic procedures after concentrated training in urological laparoscopy. *The Journal of Urology*, Vol.166, No.6, pp. 2109-2111, ISSN 1527-3792

Chou DS, Abdelshehid CS, Uribe CA, Khonsari SS, Eichel L, Boker JR, Shanberg AM, Ahlering TE, Clayman RV, McDougall EM. (2005). Initial impact of a dedicated postgraduate laparoscopic mini-residency on clinical practice patterns. *Journal of Endourology*, Vol.19, No.3, pp. 360-365, ISSN 1557-900X

Chung SY, Landsittel D, Chon CH, Ng CS, Fuchs GJ. (2005). Laparoscopic skills training using a webcam trainer. *The Journal of Urology*, Vol.173, No.1, pp. 180-183, ISSN 1527-3792

Clayman RV, Kavoussi LR, Soper NJ, Dierks SM, Merety KS, Darcy MD, Long SR, Roemer FD, Pingleton ED, Thomson PG. (1991). Laparoscopic nephrectomy. *The New England Journal of Medicine*, Vol.324, No. 19, pp. 1370-1371, ISSN 1533-4406

Colegrove PM, Winfield HN, Donovan JF, et al. Laparoscopic practice patterns among North American urologists 5 years after formal training. (1999) *The Journal of Urology*, Vol.161, No.3, pp. 881-886, ISSN 1527-3792

Corica F, Boker JR, Chou DS, White SM, Abdelshehid CS, Stoliar G, Sala LG, Shanberg AM, Clayman RV, McDougall EM. (2006) Short-term impact of a laparoscopic "mini-residency" experience on postgraduate urologists' practice patterns. *Journal of the American College of Surgeons*, Vol.203, No.3, pp.692-698, ISSN 1879-190

Cuschieri A. (1995). Whither minimal access surgery:tribulations and expectations. *American Journal of Surgery*, Vol.169, No.1, pp.9-18, ISSN 1879-1883

Dent TL. (1991). Training, credentialing, and granting of clinical privileges for laparoscopic general surgery. *American Journal of Surgery*, Vol.161, No.3, pp. 399-403, 1879-1883

Derosis AM, Fried GM, Abrahamowicz M, Sigman HH, Barkun JS, Meakins JL. (1998). Development of a model for training and evaluation of laparoscopic skills. Am *American Journal of Surgery*, Vol.175, No.6, pp. 482-487, ISSN 1879-1883

Duffy AJ, Hogle NJ, McCarthy H, Lew JI, Egan A, Christos P, Fowler DL. (2005). Construct validity for the LAPSIM laparoscopic surgical simulator. *Surgical Endoscopy*, Vol.19, No.3, pp. 401-405. ISSN 1432-2218

Emken JL, McDougall EM, Clayman RV. (2004). Training and assessment of laparoscopic skills. *Journal of the Society of Laparoendoscopic Surgeons*, Vol.8, No.2, pp. 195-199, ISSN 1938-3797

Eriksen JR, Grantcharov T. (2005) Objective assessment of laparoscopic skills using a virtual simulator. *Surgical Endoscopy*, Vol.19, No.9, pp. 1216-1219, ISSN 1432-2218

European Association of Endoscopic Surgeons. (1994). Training and assessment of competence. *Surgical Endoscopy*, Vol.8, No.6, pp. 721-722, ISSN 1432-2218

Fabrizio MD, Tuerk I, Schellhammer PF. (2003). Laparoscopic radical prostatectomy: decreasing the learning curve using a mentor initiated approach. *The Journal of Urology*, Vol.169, No.6, pp. 2063-2065, ISSN 1527-3792

Figert PL, Park AE, Witzke DB, Schwartz RW. (2001). Transfer of training in acquiring laparoscopic skills. *Journal of the American College of Surgeons*, Vol.193, No.5, pp.533-537, ISSN 1879-190

Gallagher AG, Richie K, McClure N, McGuigan J. (2001). Objective psychomotor skills assessment of experienced, junior, and novice laparoscopists with virtual reality. *World Journal of Surgery*, Vol.25, No.11, pp. 1478-1483, ISSN 1432-2323

Gaston KE, Moore DT, Pruthi RS. (2004). Hand-assisted laparoscopic nephrectomy: prospective evaluation of learning curve. *The Journal of Urology*, Vol.171, No.1, pp. 63-67, ISSN 1527-3792

Gomella LG, Strup SE. The history of urologic laparoscopy: from cystoscope to laparoscope. In Laparoscopic Urologic Surgery, Eds. Gomella LG, Kozminski M, Winfield HN. Raven Press, Ltd., New York © 1994; pp 9-14, ISBN 0781700442

Greco EF, Regher G, Okrainec. (2010). Identifying and classifying problem areas in laparoscopic skills acquisition: Can simulators help? *Academic Medicine*, Vol.85, No.10 Suppl, pp. S5-S8, ISSN 1938-808X

Hasson HM. (2006). Core competency in laparoendoscopic surgery. *Journal of the Society of Laparoendoscopic Surgeons*, Vol.10, No.1, pp. 16-20, ISSN 1938-3797

Hedican SP, Nakada SY. (2007) Videotape mentoring and surgical simulation in laparoscopic courses. *Journal of Endourology*, Vol.21, No.3, pp. 288-293, ISSN 1557-900X

Higashihara E, Baba S, Nakagawa K, Murai M, Go H, Takeda M, Takahashi K, Suzuki K, Fujita K, Yoshinari O, Ohshima S, Matsuda T, Terachi T, Yoshida O. (1998). Learning curve and conversion to open surgery in cases of laparoscopic adrenalectomy and nephrectomy. *The Journal of Urology*, Vol.159, No.3, pp.650-653, ISSN 1527-3792

Hollenbeck BK, Seifman BD, Wolf JS Jr. (2004). Clinical skills acquisition for hand-assisted laparoscopic donor nephrectomy. *The Journal of Urology*, Vol.171, No.1, pp.35-39, ISSN 1527-3792

Hoznek A, Salomon L, de la Taille A, Yiou R, Vordos D, Larre S, Abbou CC. (2006). Simulation training in video-assisted urologic surgery. *Current Urology Reports*, Vol.171, No.1. pp.107-113, ISSN 1534-6285

Hruza M, Weib HO, Pini G, Goezen AS, Schulze M, Teber D, Rassweiler JJ. (2010). Complications in 2200 consecutive laparoscopic radical prostatectomies: standardized evaluation and analysis of learning curves. *European Urology*, Vol.58, No.5, pp.733-741, ISSN 1873-7560

Jeon SH, Han K, Yoo KH, Choe BK, Seo IY, Lim JS, Ono Y. (2009). How many cases are necessary to develop competence for laparoscopic radical nephrectomy? *Journal of Endourology*, Vol.23, No.12, pp.1965-1970, ISSN 1557-900X

Katz R, Hoznek A, Antiphon P, Van Velthoven R, Delmas V, Abbou CC. (2003). Cadaveric versus porcine models in urologic laparoscopic training. *Urologia Internationalis*, Vol.71, No.3, pp.310-315, 1423-0399

Katz R, Hoznek A, Salomon L, Antiphon P, de la Taille A, Abbou CC. (2005). Skill assessment of urologic surgeons: Can criterion levels of surgical performance be determined using the pelvic box trainer? *European Urology*, Vol.47, No.4, pp. 47:482-487, ISSN 1873-7560

Kavic MS. (2002). Competency and the six core competencies. JSLS, Vol.6, No.2, pp. 95-97.

Kolla SB, Gamboa AJ, Li R, Santos RT, Gan JM, Shell C, Andrade L, Louie MK, Clayman RV,

McDougall EM. (2010). Impact of a laparoscopic renal surgery mini-fellowship program on postgraduate urologist practice patterns at a 3-year follow-up. *The Journal of Urology*, Vol.184, No.5, pp.2089-2093, ISSN 1527-3792

Kumar U, Gill IS. (2006). Learning curve in human laparoscopic surgery. *Current Urology Reports*, Vol.7, No.2, pp. 120-124, ISSN 1534-6285Link RE, Bhayani SB, Allaf ME, Varkarakis I, Inagaki T, Rodgers C, Su L, Jarrett TW,

Kavoussi LR. (2005). Exploring the learning curve, pathological outcomes and perioperative morbidity of laparoscopic partial nephrectomy performed for renal mass. *The Journal of Urology*, Vol.173, No.5, pp. 1690-1694, ISSN 1527-3792

Laguna MP, de Reijke TM, Wijkstra H, de la Rosette J. (2006). Training in laparoscopic urology. *Current Opinion in Urology*, Vol.16, No.2, pp.65-70, ISSN 1473-6586

Lynch J, Aughwane P, Hammond TM. (2010). Video games and surgical ability:A literature review. *Journal of Surgical Education*, Vol.67, No.3, pp. 184-189, 1878-7452

McDougall EM. (2007). Validation of surgical simulators. *Journal of Endourology*, Vol.21, No.3, pp.244-247, ISSN 1557-900X

Maithel S, Sierra R, Korndorffer J, Neumann P, Dawson S, Callery M, Jones D, Scott D. (2006). Construct and face validity of MIST-VR, Endotower and CELTS: Are we ready for skills assessment using simulators? *Surgical Endoscopy*, Vol.20, No.1, pp.104-112, ISSN 1432-2218

Marguet CG, Young MD, L'Esperance JO, Tan YH, Ekeruo WO, Preminger GM, Albala DM. (2004). Hand assisted laparoscopic training for postgraduate urologists:The role of mentoring. *The Journal of Urology*, Vol.172, No.1, pp.286-289, ISSN 1527-3792

Martin JA, Regehr G, Reznick R, MacRae H, Murnaghan J, Hutchinson C, Brown M. (1997). Objective structured assessment of technical skill (OSATS) for surgical residents. *The British Journal of Surgery*, Vol.84, No.2, pp. 273-278, ISSN 0007-1323

Munver R, Del Pizzo JJ, Sosa RE. (2004). The advantages of hand-assisted laparoscopy. *Current Urology Reports*, Vol.5, No.2, pp.100-7, ISSN 1534-6285

Nakada SY, Moon TD, Gist M, Mahvi D. (1997). Use of the pneumo sleeve as an adjunct in laparoscopic nephrectomy. *Urology*, Vol.49, No.4, pp. 612-613, ISSN 1527-9995

Nakada SY, Hedican SP, Bishoff JT, Shichman SJ, Wolf JS Jr. (2004). Expert videotape analysis and critiquing benefit laparoscopic skills training of urologists. *Journal of the Society of Laparoendoscopic Surgeons*, Vol.8, No.2, pp.183-186, ISSN 1938-3797

Nelson CP, Wolf JS Jr. (2002). Comparison of hand-assisted versus standard laparoscopic radical nephrectomy for suspected renal cell carcinoma. *The Journal of Urology*, Vol.167, No.5, pp.1989-1994, ISSN 1527-3792

Pareek G, Hedican SP, Bishoff JT, Shichman SJ, Wolf JS Jr, Nakada SY. (2008). Skills-based laparoscopy training demonstrates long-term transfer of clinical laparoscopic practice:additional follow-up. *Urology*, No.72, No.2, pp.265-267, ISSN 1527-9995

Phillips J, Catto JW, Lavin V, Doyle D, Smith DJ, Hastie KJ, Oakley NE. (2005). The laparoscopic nephrectomy learning curve: a single centre's development of a de novo practice. *Postgraduate Medical Journal*, Vol.81, No.959, pp.599-603, ISSN 1469-0756

Piechaud PT, Pansadoro A. (2006). Transfer of skills from the experimental model to the patients. *Current Urology Reports*, Vol.7, No.2, pp.96-99, ISSN 1534-6285

Pietrow PK, Auge BK, Terranova S, Ekeruo W, Preminger GM, Albala DM. (2004). Hand-assisted laparoscopic nephrectomy:the transfer of experience to a new academic center. *Journal of Endourology*, Vol.18, No.9, pp. 840-843, ISSN 1557-900X

Rane A. (2005). A training module for laparoscopic urology. JSLS, Vol.9, No.4, pp.460-462.

Rassweiler J, Klein J, Teber D, Schulze M, Frede T. (2007). Mechanical simulators for training for laparoscopic surgery in urology. *Journal of Endourology*, Vol.21, No.3, pp.252-262, ISSN 1557-900X

Ratner LE, Cisek LJ, Moore RG, Cigarroa FG, Kaufman HS, Kavoussi LR. (1995). Laparoscopic live donor nephrectomy. *Transplantation*, Vol.60, No.9, pp.1047-1049, ISSN 0041-1337

Rawlins MC, Hefty TL, Brown SL, Biehl TR. (2002). Learning laparoscopic donor nephrectomy safely: a report on 100 cases. Arch Surg, Vol.137, No.5, pp.531-535.

Rosser JC, Lynch PJ, Cuddihy L, Gentile DA, Klonsky J, Merrell R. (2007). The impact of video games on training surgeons in the 21st century. *Archives of Surgery*, Vol.142, No.2, pp.181-186, ISSN 0272-5533

Scott DJ, Young WN, Tesfay ST, Frawley WH, Rege RV, Jones DB. (2001). Laparoscopic skills training. *American Journal of Surgery*, Vol.182, No.2, pp.137-142, ISSN 1879-1883

Secin FP, Savage C, Abbou C, de la Taille A, Saloman L, Rassweiler J, Hruza M, Rozet F, Cathelineaux X, Janetschek G, NAssar F, Turk I, Vanni AJ, Gill IS, Koenig P, Kaouk JH, Pineiro LM, Pansadoro V, Emiliozzi P, Bjartell A, Jiborn T, Eden C, Richards AJ, Van Velthoven R, Stolzenberg J, Rabenalt R, Su L, Pavlovish CP, Levinson AW, Touijer KA, Vikers A, Guillonneau B. (2010). The learning curve for laparoscopic radical prostatectomy: an international multicenter study. *The Journal of Urology*, Vol.184, No.6, pp.2291-2296, ISSN 1527-3792

See WA, Cooper CS, Fisher RJ. (1994). Urological laparoscopic practice patterns 1 year after formal training. *The Journal of Urology*, Vol.151, No.6, pp.1595-1598, ISSN 1527-3792

Seymour NE, Gallagher AB, Roman SA, O'Brien MK, Bansal VK, Andersen DK, Satava RM. (2002). Virtual reality training improves operating room performance:results of a randomized, double-blinded study. *Annals of Surgery*, Vol.236, No.4, pp.458-463, ISSN 0003-4932

Shalhav AL, Dabagia MD, Wagner TT, Koch MO, Lingeman JE. (2002). Training postgraduate urologists in laparoscopic surgery: the current challenge. *The Journal of Urology*, Vol.167, No.5, pp.2135-2137, ISSN 1527-3792

Smith CD, Farrell TM, McNatt SS, Metreveli RE. (2001). Assessing laparoscopic manipulative skills. *American Journal of Surgery*, Vol.181, No.6, pp.547-550, ISSN 1879-1883

Smith SG, Torkington J, Brown TJ, Taffinder NJ, Darzi A. (2002). Motion analysis. *Surgical Endoscopy*, Vol.16, No.4, pp.640-645, ISSN 1432-2218

Stelzer MK, Abdel MP, Sloan MP, Gould JC. (2009). Dry lab practice leads to improved laparoscopic performance in the operating room. *The Journal of Surgical Research*, Vol.154, No.1, pp.163-166, ISSN 1095-8673

Szinicz G, Beller S, Bodner W, Zerz A, Szincz S. (2001). Simulated operations by pulsatile organ-perfusion in minimally invasive surgery. *Surgical Laparoscopy & Endoscopy*, Vol.15, No.4, pp. 232-241, ISSN 1051-7200

Taffinder NJ, Smith SG, Mair J, Russell RC, Darzi A. (1999). Can a computer measure surgical precision? Reliability, validity and feasibility of the ICSAD. *Surgical Endoscopy*, Vol.13, No.Suppl 1, pp.S81, ISSN 1432-2218

Taffinder N, Sutton C, Fishwick RJ, McManus IC, Darzi A. (1998). Validation of virtual reality to teach and assess psychomotor skills in laparoscopic surgery: results from randomized controlled studies using the MIST VR laparoscopic simulator. *Studies in Health Technology and Informatics*, Vol.50, pp.124-130, ISSN 0926-9630

Thijssen AS, Schijven MP. (2010). Contemporary virtual reality laparoscopy simulators: quicksand or solid grounds for assessing surgical trainees? *American Journal of Surgery*, Vol.199, No.4, pp.529-541, ISSN 1879-1883

Torkington J, Smith SG, Rees BI, Darzi A. (2001). Skill transfer from virtual reality to a real laparoscopic task. *Surgical Endoscopy*, Vol.15, No.10, pp.1076-1079, ISSN 1432-2218

Undre S, Darzi A. (2007). Laparoscopy simulators. J Endourol, Vol.21, No.3, pp.274-279.

Vlaovic PD, Sargent ER, Boker JR, Corica FA, Chou DS, Abdelshehid CS, White SM, Sala LG, Chu F, Le T, Clayman RV, McDougall EM. (2008). Immediate impact of an intensive one-week laparoscopy training program on laparoscopic skills among postgraduate urologists. *Journal of the Society of Laparoendoscopic Surgeons*, Vol.12, No.1, pp.1-8, ISSN 1938-3797

Wignall GR, Denstedt JD, Preminger GM, Cadeddu JA, Pearle MS, Sweet RM, McDougall EM. (2008). Surgical simulation: A urological perspective. *The Journal of Urology*, Vol.179, No.5, pp.1690-1699, ISSN 1527-3792

Part 2

Surgery

Laparoscopic Adrenalectomy

Craig N Parnaby and Patrick J O'Dwyer
University of Glasgow, Glasgow
United Kingdom

1. Introduction

Laparoscopic adrenalectomy (LA) was first described by Gagner et al in 1992 (Gagner et al., 1992). Since this time LA has become the procedure of choice for most adrenal pathologies. Multiple case-control studies have consistently demonstrated the benefits of LA compared to open adrenalectomy (OA) in terms of blood loss, analgesic requirments, postoperative complications, hospital stay and earlier return to normal activity.

2. Clinical presentation

Clinical presentation can often be non-specific or the patient can present after incidental adrenal gland imaging.

2.1 Conn's syndrome

Conn's syndrome is an aldosterone producing adenoma. The symptoms and signs are non-specific and include hypertension and hypokalaemia.

2.2 Cushing's syndrome

Symptoms and signs are related to excess cortisol production. These include: truncal obesity, decreased libido, thin skin, hypertension, hirsutism, depression, easy bruising, glucose intolerance and general weakness.

2.3 Phaeochromocytoma

A phaeochromocytoma is usually associated with excess production of catecholamines. The tumour can be suspected when a patient presents with: episodic episodes of headaches, sweating and palpitations with poorly controlled persistent or intermittent hypertension.

2.4 Incidentaloma

Adrenal incidentaloma is an adrenal tumour (≥1cm) discovered on an imaging study for other unrelated pathologies. Over the last one and a half decades incidental adrenal gland imaging is increasingly performed as computed tomography for other abdominal pathologies has become common. This has led to an increase in patients with an incidental adrenal tumour referred for surgical and endocrine assessment (Saunders et al., 2004). Presently between 4-6% of the imaged population have incidentalomas (Bovio et al., 2006; Kloos et al., 1995). Almost all these lesions will be benign in a patient without a known history of cancer (Song et al., 2007; Young, 2000).

2.5 Adrenal metastasis

Adrenal metastasis should be considered in any patient with known extraadrenal malignancy and an isolated adrenal lesion >2cm or an adrenal mass increasing in size on serial imaging (Bonnet et al.,2008).

3. Assessment of adrenal tumours

Adrenal tumours are characterised by radiological and hormonal assessment.

3.1 Hormonal assessment

All adrenal tumours require a hormone evaluation. The hormone studies are performed to check for: phaeochromocytoma, hypercortisolism and hyperaldosteronism. However, there is no consensus regarding the best hormone diagnostic approach.

A suggested approach would be:

1. A phaeochromocytoma screen included a 24 hour urine collection for catecholamines (norepinephrine, epinephrine and dopamine) and metabolites (metanephrine, normetanephrine, vanillylmandelic acid).
2. Hypercortisolism assessment included an overnight dexamethasone suppression test. If positive a suppressed morning plasma ACTH and DHEAS level can be used to support the diagnosis (Nieman, 2010).
3. Hyperaldosteronism should be excluded in hypertensive patients. A screen included urea and electrolytes, plasma aldosterone-to-renin ratio. Adrenal vein sampling can be used for patients with suspected Conn's syndrome when imaging does not demonstrate an obvious adenoma.

3.2 Radiological assessment

The main modalities of choice in the evaluation of an adrenal tumour are computed tomography (CT) or magnetic resonance imaging (MRI). Most investigators use CT as the initial modality of choice as it is readily available and cheaper. Occasionally when CT or MRI studies are inconclusive patients are referred for combined positron emission tomography and computed tomography (PET-CT).

Adrenal tumours can be characterized using imaging alone. Characterisation of the adrenal tumour depends on a number of factors which include: morphology, perfusion differences and intracellular lipid concentration (Boland et al., 2008).

Morphology appearances which may suggest malignancy include: increased size, large necrotic areas, increased heterogeneity, irregular borders and local invasion. Available data suggests, at a size threshold of ≥4cm the likelihood of malignancy doubles and is more than ninefold higher for tumours ≥8cm (Sturgeon et al., 2006).

Lipid sensitive imaging by CT or MRI exploit the fact that most adenomas contain abundant intracellular fat where as almost all malignant lesions do not (Korobkin et al., 1996). It has been reported an unenhanced CT densitometry technique can effectively differentiate many adrenal adenomas from malignant adenomas. Figure 3.1 shows a typical adrenal adenoma from an unenhanced CT.

If the CT attenuation threshold is set at 10 hounsfield units the sensitivity and specificity for characterising adenomas versus non-adenomas has been reported 71% and 98% respectively (Boland et al.,1998). This method has limitations which include: up to 30 % of adenomas are lipid poor and most CT scans for other pathologies are contrast enhanced (Boland et al., 2008). Therefore, using attenuation values in these cases would be considered indeterminate or difficult to interpret.

More recently studies have reported improved results using CT perfusion washout scans or chemical shift MR imaging. For CT, an initial non-contrast or contrast enhanced scan is performed followed by a contrast enhanced examination after a variable delay (often 15 minutes). Benign lesions typically demonstrate more than 50% washout. A threshold enhancement washout value is then calculated. Chemical shift MR imaging utilises the different resonant frequencies of fat and water protons. Benign lesions typically show signal intensity decrease when compared with in-phase images. From the available data, CT perfusion washout scan appears to offer the highest sensitivity and specificity for adrenal adenoma characterization (Park et al., 2007).

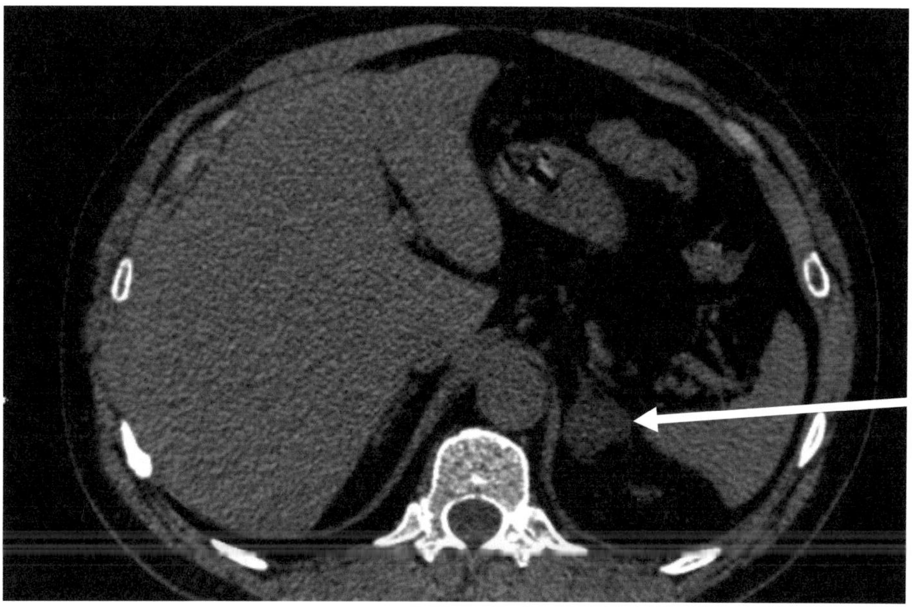

Fig. 3.1 Unenhanced CT of a left adrenal adenoma (arrow)

PET-CT allows adrenal lesion morphology and metabolic activity to be coregistered on the same image. This would allow a more accurate anatomic localization of any PET abnormalities. In current practice patients would only be referred for PET-CT rarely if CT or MR results are inconclusive (Boland et al., 2008).

^{123}I-MIBG is concentrated in catecholamine storage vesicles. A meta-iodobenzylguanidine (MIBG) scan can help identify phaeochromocytoma, extra-adrenal phaeochromocytoma and metastatic deposits from the phaeochromocytoma.

Despite the above techniques, the only reliable imaging findings to differentiate between malignant and benign adrenal tumours remain the presence of regional invasion or metastatic disease.

3.3 Adrenal fine-needle aspiration (FNA)

Ultrasound or computed tomography guided FNA is unhelpful to distinguish between benign and malignant adrenal tumours due to the high false negative rate (Sasano et al.,1995). The only potential use of FNA is to help diagnose metastasis when adrenal resection is not planned and detection would alter patient management (Lee et al., 1998).

3.4 Suggested hormonal and radiological approach to an adrenal tumour

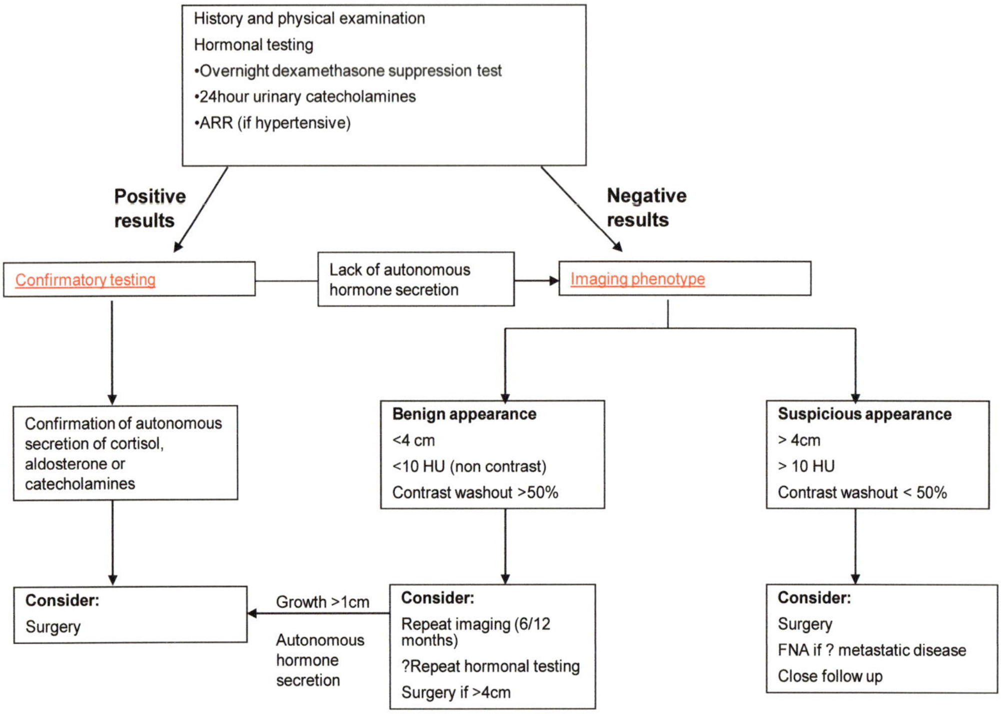

Fig. 3.2 gives a suggested algorithm for the evaluation of an adrenal tumour

4. Indication for adrenalectomy

Adrenalectomy is indicated for all hormonally active adrenal lesions, suspicion of adrenal malignancy on imaging (size ≥4cm, local invasion, tumour heterogeneity, high attenuation and irregular tumour margins) and isolated adrenal metastases. Resection of non functioning adrenal tumours <4cm was indicated for patients with evidence of tumour growth on serial radiological imaging.

Management of a non functioning adrenal lesion remains debatable. All authors advocate resection of large ≥6cm non functional adrenal tumours due to the increased risk of malignancy. No prospective controlled studies exist for the role of adrenalectomy for adrenal masses of 3-6 cm. Different authors have advocated size tumour thresholds of 3,4,5 and 6cm for resection of non functioning adrenal tumours (Duh, 2002; Thompson et al., 2003; Eldeiry & Garber, 2008). Sturgeon et al characterized the relationship between tumour size and malignancy risk compared the National Cancer Institute's Surveillance, Epidemiology, and End Results (SEER) database for adrenocortical carcinoma with their own experience with benign adrenal cortical adenomas from a similar time period. From the SEER database 457 adrenal cortical carcinomas were identified (376 had size data) and 47 patients from their own series with benign adrenal cortical adenomas. The authors found a tumour threshold of 4cm has a sensitivity and specificity of 96% and 52% for malignancy versus 90% and 80% for a tumour threshold of 6cm. The authors advocated that all tumours ≥4cm should be surgical resected (Sturgeon et al., 2006).

4.1 Indications for laparoscopic adrenalectomy

Within a specialised centre, we feel the only contraindication to laparoscopy were large locally invasive adrenal carcinoma or the requirement of an additional open operation.

5. Perioperative management

5.1 Bilateral adrenalectomy

Bilateral adrenalectomy can be indicated following relapse after pituitary surgery, bilateral adrenal hyperplasia or hereditary phaeochromocytoma. Perioperative intravenous hydrocortisone is required to prevent acute adrenal insufficiency. When oral intake has been established lifelong oral steroids are required. Increased doses are required at times of stress (eg trauma, infection).

5.2 Autonomous cortisol secretion

For patients with autonomous cortisol secretion after hormonal testing a perioperative 'stress dose' of hydrocortisone is recommended. A post operative in-patient short SYNACTHEN test would follow. If the test indicates adrenal insufficiency (low level of stimulated cortisol) steroid replacement should continue as this indicates hypothalamic-pituitary-adrenal (HPA) axis suppression. Patients are then reviewed as an out-patient to test for HPA axis recovery. If the test indicates adequate cortisol response (functioning HPA axis) steroid replacement therapy can stop.

5.3 Phaeochromocytoma

The perioperative medical management of patients with phaeochromocytomas is essential to reduce the effects of circulating catecholamines (Plouin et al., 2001; Kinney et al., 2000). These can include severe hypertension (systolic blood pressure >200mmHg), tachycardia, arrhythmias and death. Immediate surgery is rarely essential.

Medical management aims to control blood pressure, heart rate and arrhythmias. Traditional preoperative regimens have included phenoxybenzamine (a long-acting non-selective alpha blocker) and propanolol (beta blocker) (Ross et al., 1967). Other agents have been used effectively including selective alpha blockers and calcium channel antagonists (Prys-Roberts & Farndon., 2002; Lebuffe et al., 2005). No randomised trial exists comparing the traditional regimen with other medical managements. Currently, the most effective perioperative drug regimen for patients undergoing phaeochromocytoma resection is unknown.

Despite preoperative medical management, intraoperative tumour manipulation or introduction of pneumoperitoneum (laparoscopic adrenalectomy) may cause severe haemodynamic responses requiring further treatment with short acting alpha blockers (eg phentolamine) or short acting beta blockers (eg labetalol) (Joris et al., 1999; Tauzin-Fin et al., 2004).

The current regimen we use at the Western Infirmary, Glasgow, is as follows. At initial endocrine assessment, all patients with a suspected phaeochromocytoma received oral phenoxybenzamine as the primary alpha blocker (range 10-60mg/day). This was titrated to achieve a blood pressure measurement <160/90 mmHg. Patients were not routinely beta-blocked in the preoperative period. Hypertension was controlled in all phaeochromocytoma patients prior to elective resection.

All patients in the phaeochromocytoma group received an infusion of phenoxybenzamine (1mg kg^{-1}, a non selective long acting alpha blocker) the day before LA. Oral phenoxybenzamine was discontinued the day before theatre.

Arterial blood pressure is monitored using a radial arterial line. During surgery, episodes of hypertension (SBP>180mmHg) were treated with intravenous phentolamine (boluses 1 to 2mg) and/or labetalol (boluses 5 to 10mg). Tachycardia was treated with intravenous labetalol (boluses 5 to 10mg). Hypotension was treated with fluid boluses (crystalloid or colloid) and/or an intravenous vasopressor (metaraminol).

There is some concern that the persistent α-adrenoceptor blockade caused by phenoxybenzamine after resection can cause persistent hypotension resistant to adrenergic arteriolar constrictors and large volumes of intravascular fluid (Prys-Roberts et al., 2002). This has not been realised in our series. From January 1999 - January 2009, there were 42 consecutive LA performed for phaeochromocytoma. No patient experienced persistent hypotension (systolic blood pressure <80mmHg >10 minutes) in the recovery room period.

6. Laparoscopic adrenalectomy

Laparoscopic adrenalectomy was first described by Gagner et al in 1992 (Gagner et al., 1992). They described a successful anterior transabdominal approach in 3 patients (Cushing's syndrome, Cushing's disease and a phaeochromocytoma). The authors felt that LA may reduce morbidity, reduce analgesic requirements and reduce post operative stay when compared to open adrenalectomy (OA).

Since this time, multiple case-control studies have consistently demonstrated the benefits of LA compared OA in terms of blood loss, analgesic requirements, post operative complications, hospital stay and earlier return to normal activity for a variety of adrenal gland pathologies. Table 6.1 gives an overview of outcomes for studies comparing LA versus OA.

Despite the lack of Level 1 evidence comparing LA with OA, it seems unlikely randomized controlled trials will be performed. This is primarily due to the benefits consistently demonstrated in favour of LA.

Therefore, LA has become the procedure of choice for most adrenal gland pathologies in high-volume centres.

6.1 Laparoscopic operative technique

Laparoscopic approaches to the adrenal gland include the lateral transabdominal approach, the retroperitoneal approach or the anterior transabdominal approach.

The lateral transabdominal approach is the most popular approach in published case series. Reasons include: easiest to learn due to presence of an increased number of anatomical landmarks compared to the retroperitoneal approach and the ability to perform large adrenal tumour (≥6cm) resection.

The retroperitoneal approach was first described in 1995 (Mercan et al., 1995) and subsequent series have since reported a safety and efficacy comparable to other laparoscopic approaches (Hanssen et al., 2006; Bonjer et al.,2000; Walz et al., 2006). Potential drawbacks to this approach include lack of familiarity amongst most general surgeons, limited working

Author	Year	No. of patients		Blood loss (mls)*		Analgesia requirements	Complications (%)		Length of stay (days)*	
		LA	OA	LA	OA	(LA versus OA)	LA	OA	LA	OA
(Brunt et al., 1996))	1996	24	42	104 387		Reduced analgesia requirement	17	64	3.2	7.5
(MacGillivray, Shichman, Ferrer, & Malchoff, 1996)	1996	17	12	198 500		n.a	21	56	3	7.9
(Staren & Prinz, 1996)	1996	21	20	n.a.		n.a.	n.a.		2.2	6.1
(G. B. Thompson et al., 1997)	1997	50	50	n.a.		Reduced analgesia requirement	6	72	3.1	5.7
(Jacobs, Goldstein, & Geer, 1997)	1997	19	19	109 263		n.a.	5	38	2.3	5.1
(Linos et al., 1997)	1997	18	147	n.a.		Reduced duration of PCA use	0	12	2.2	6.3
(Vargas et al., 1997)	1997	20	20	245 283		Reduced analgesia requirement	10	25	3.1	7.2
(Winfield, Hamilton, Bravo, & Novick, 1998)	1998	21	17	183 266		Reduced analgesia requirement	29	76	2.7	6.2
(Ting, Lo, & Lo, 1998)	1998	12	56	50 150		Reduced analgesia requirement	0	9	3	5
(Imai, Kikumori, Ohiwa, Mase, & Funahashi, 1999)	1999	40	40	40 172		Reduced analgesia requirement	5	50	12	18
(Dudley & Harrison, 1999)	1999	36	23	n.a.		n.a.	6	52	3.5	8.5
(Soares, Monchik, Migliori, & Amaral, 1999)	1999	12	7	132 278		Reduced analgesia requirement	8	0	2.1	5.4
(Schell, Talamini, & Udelsman, 1999)	1999	22	17	n.a.		n.a.	n.a.		1.7	6.7
(Shen et al., 1999)	1999	42	38	n.a.		n.a.	0	11	n.a.	
(Rayan & Hodin, 2000)	2000	19	48	n.a.		n.a.	3	60	1.5	6.3
(Hazzan et al., 2001)	2001	24	28	n.a.		Reduced analgesia requirement	16	39	4	7.5
(Ortega, Sala, Garcia, & Lledo, 2002)	2002	10	10	n.a.		n.a.	10	30	3.7	5.8

*Values are mean. LA, laparoscopic adrenalectomy; OA, open adrenalectomy;
PCA, patient controlled analgesia;n.a., data not available

Table 6.1. Outcomes for laparoscopic adrenalectomy versus open adrenalectomy

space and the unsuitability for resection of large adrenal tumours (≥6cm). Potential advantages include: avoidance of the peritoneal cavity in patients with previous upper gastrointestinal surgery and no need to change position in bilateral adrenalectomy (if prone jackknife position used). From available studies, patient outcome remains similar compared to the lateral transabdominal approach for small-medium sized tumours.
The anterior transabdominal approach is practised infrequently and therefore the evidence favouring this approach is scarce. The main reason for its unpopularity is the increased dissection, adjacent structure retraction difficulties and longer operating times compared to other procedures.
In summary, the lateral transabdominal approach is favoured by most surgeons (including the current authors) followed by the retroperitoneal approach. Both techniques will be described in detail.

6.1.1 Lateral transabdominal laparoscopic adrenalectomy

Patient positioning

The patient placed is in the lateral decubitus position with the operative side up. The table is broken to increase the space between the costal margin and iliac crest.

Left side

Step 1. Port placement
The port placements are illustrated in Figure 6.1. The middle port (10mm) is for a 30° camera and inserted using an open technique at a point just lateral to the rectus at the level of the umbilicus (a veress needle technique is an acceptable alternative). Two instrument ports (5mm, 5mm) are inserted under direct vision. One 5mm port is inserted parallel to the costal margin in the mid-clavicular line. The other 5mm port is inserted under the eleventh rib in the mid-axillary line. A further 5mm port is occasionally required to assist with splenic retraction.

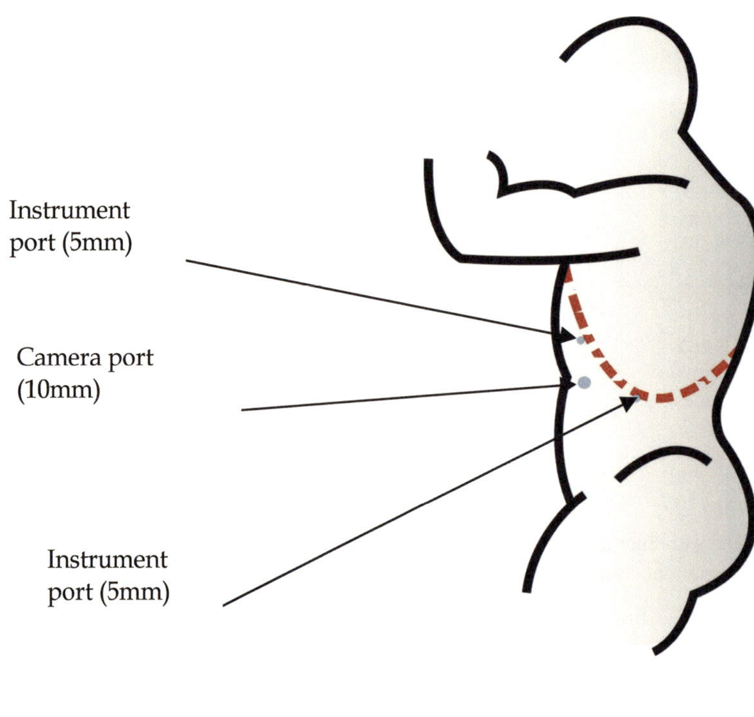

Step 2. Splenic flexure and spleen mobilisation
We use ultrasonic dissection to mobilise the splenic flexure of the colon and the lienorenal ligament of the spleen. The colon can then be displaced inferiorly and the spleen displaced medially (Figure 6.2). This allows access to the superior pole of the kidney and the adrenal gland.

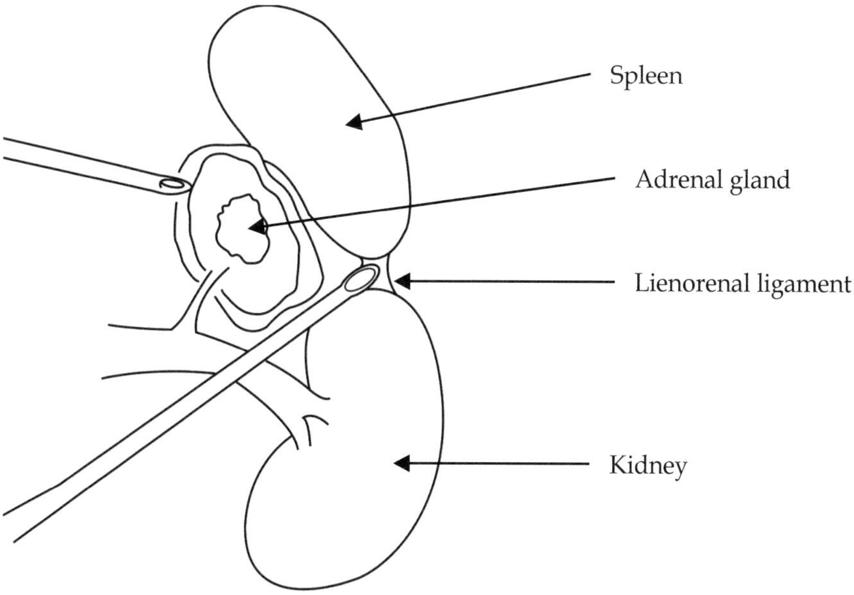

Step 3. Adrenal vein identification and division
Gerota's fascia is then opened to expose the periadrenal fat. Dissection starts at the infero-medial aspect to allow early visualisation of the left renal and then the left adrenal vein (Figure 6.3). The adrenal vein is then divided between clips. Care is taken to ensure there is no duplicate main adrenal vein.

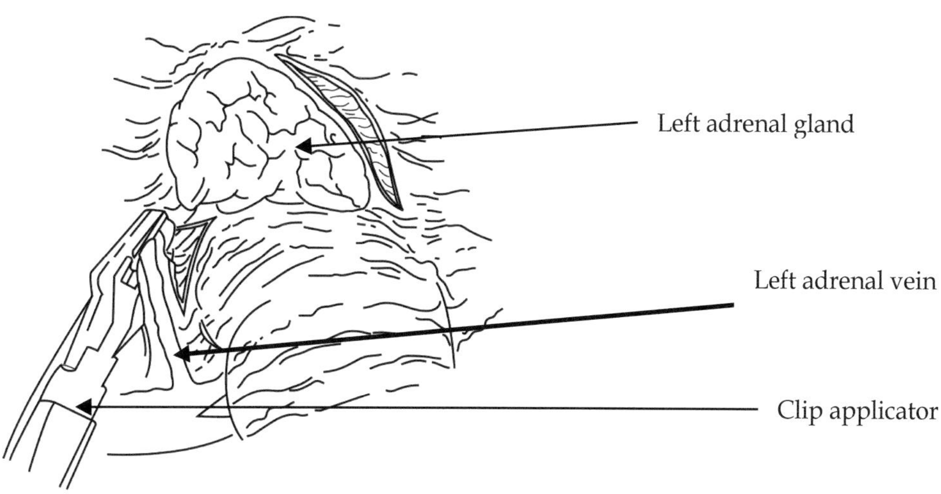

Step 4. Adrenal gland mobilisation
Avoid grasping the adrenal gland directly as it is fragile and will tear. The adrenal gland together with its surrounding fat are mobilised using ultrasonic dissection from its superior, lateral and posterior attachments. Multiple small adrenal arteries and veins will be encountered and these can all usually be divided using the harmonic scalpel.
Step 5. Adrenal gland removal
The adrenal gland is then removed via the camera port using an impermeable retrieval bag. The wound may require extension to allow retrieval.

Right side

Step 1. Port placement
The port placements are illustrated in Figure 6.4. The camera port (10mm) is inserted just lateral to the rectus at the level of the umbilicus (30° laparoscope). Two 5mm instrument ports are placed as for the left side and a third is placed in the right iliac fossa. The most medial port is used to retract the right liver lobe. We have found an atraumatic grasper offers reasonable retraction.

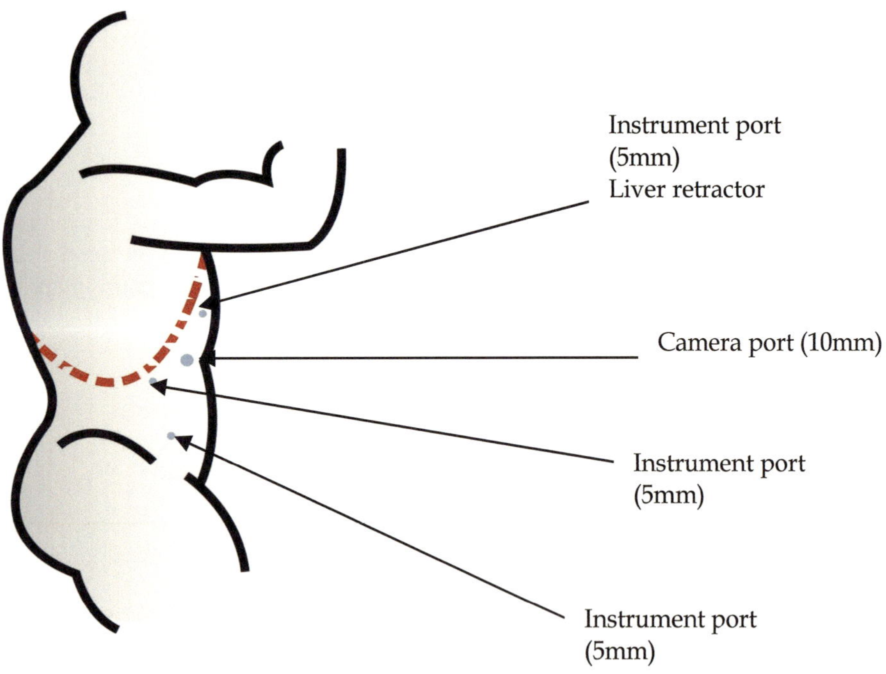

Step 2. Right liver lobe mobilisation
The right lobe of liver is mobilised from its lateral and posterior attachments and retracted (Figure 6.5). This allows access to the adrenal gland and inferior vena cava.

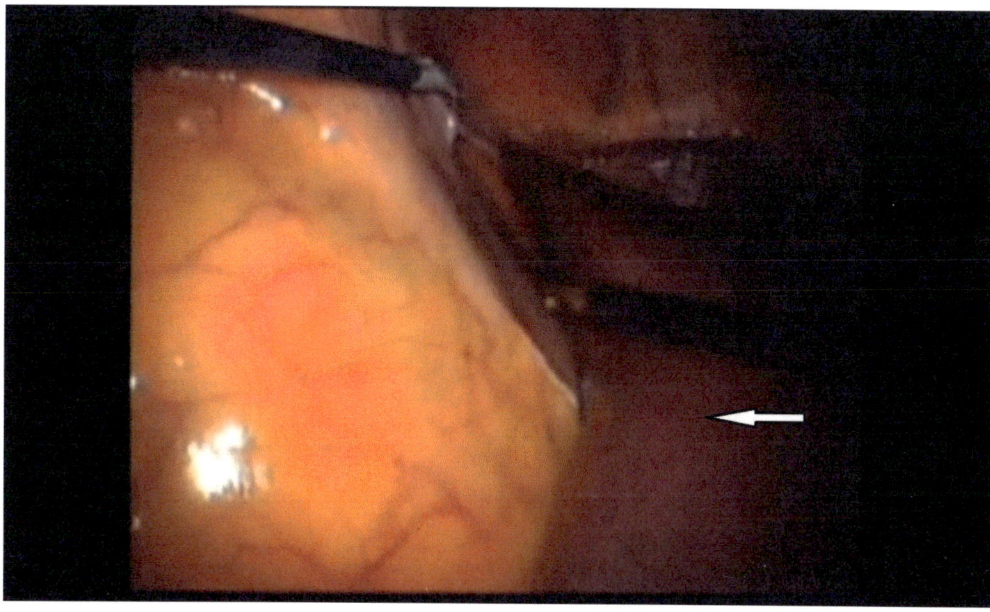

Step 3. Inferior vena cava and right adrenal vein
The peritoneum overlying the lateral edge of the inferior vena cava is divided carefully. The lateral border of the inferior vena cava is dissected from the inferior part of the liver to the origin of the right renal vein. The short main adrenal vein will be located between these points. After careful dissection the adrenal vein is divided between clips (Figure 6.6). Care should be taken as occasionally there can be a duplicate main adrenal vein.

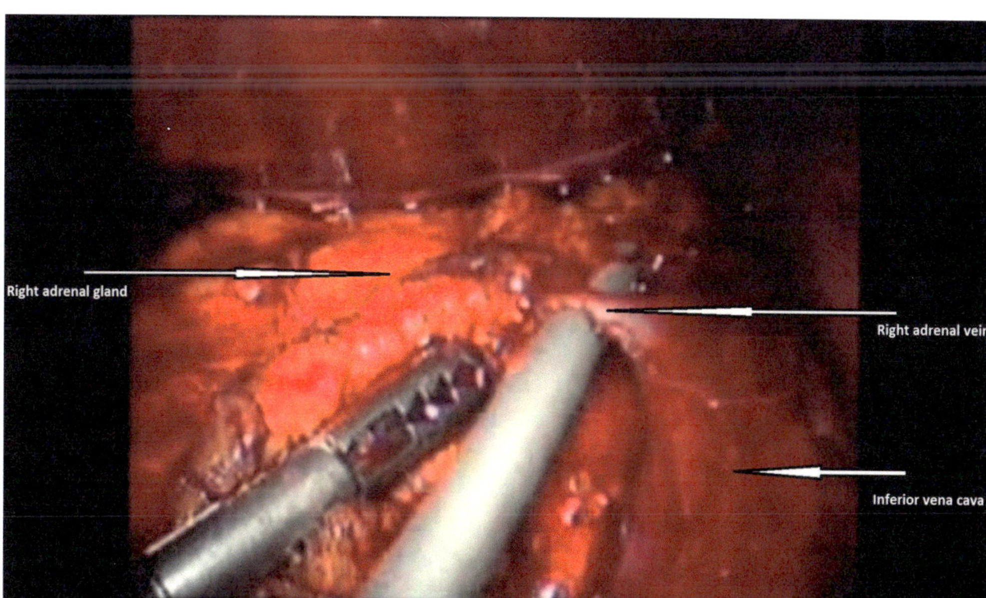

Step 4. Adrenal gland mobilisation
The adrenal gland together with its surrounding fat is then completely mobilised using ultrasonic dissection (Figure 6.7).

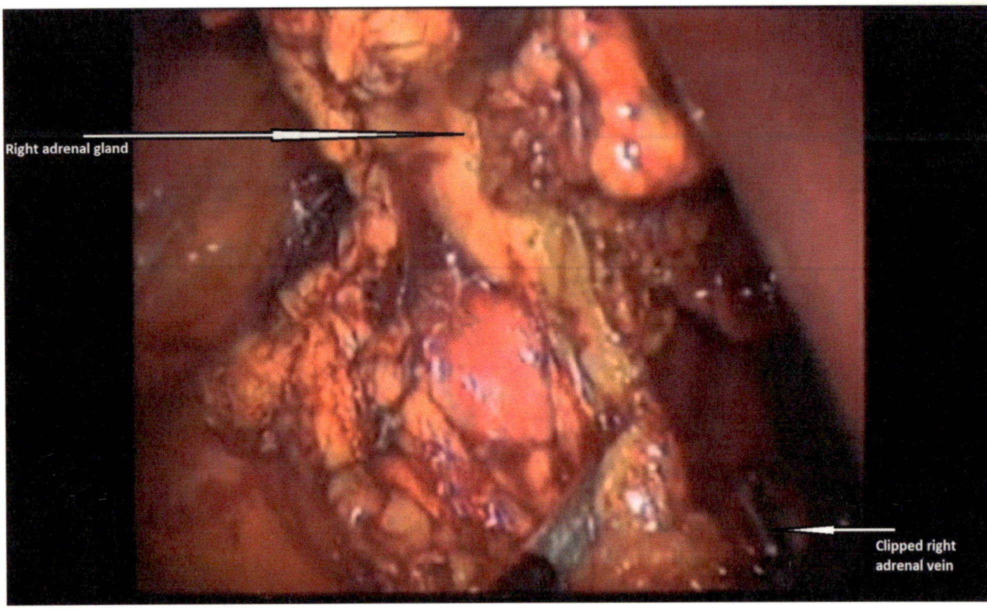

Step 5. Step 5 Adrenal gland removal
The adrenal gland and tumour is removed in the same manner as for left adrenalectomy.

6.1.2 Lateral transabdominal technique modifications for larger adrenal tumours

The laparoscopic technique was modified for large adrenal tumours. On the right side, initial dissection of the inferior vena cava and the adrenal vein is often impossible due to tumour size. We like other authors (Henry et al.,2002) start dissecting laterally, superiorly and inferiorly (often alternating between these sites). This progressive mobilisation then allows access to the inferior vena cava and the procedure continues as described above. Similarly, on the left, initial adrenal vein dissection may not be possible due to tumour size. Primary lateral, superior, inferior dissection and mobilisation allows access to the adrenal vein. Often, it is not possible to insert these large tumours into a retrieval bag. In these cases a wound protector is inserted and the tumour is removed directly through the wound.

6.1.3 Retroperitoneal laparoscopic adrenalectomy

The following operative technique has been described and then developed by Walz and colleagues (Barczynski et al.,2007).

Patient position

Patient is placed in the prone jackknife position

Left side

Step 1. Port placement
The initial 10-12mm camera port is placed using an open technique just below the 12th rib. The retroperitoneum was accessed by digital perforation of Gerota's fascia. A 30°

laparoscope was inserted and the retroperitoneal cavity was bluntly gently enlarged. Two 5mm ports were inserted, 4-5cm either side of the camera port. The retroperitoneal pressure was set at 20-25mmHg.

Step 2. Creation of a retroperitoneal space

A large retroperitoneal space is created using blunt dissection with the laparoscope and blunt dissectors. The adrenal gland tumour and upper pole of the kidney are identified.

Step 3. Initial adrenal gland mobilisation

The upper pole of the kidney is mobilised this allows access to the lower part of the adrenal gland. The inferomedial border of the adrenal gland is then carefully mobilised.

Step 4. Identification and division of main adrenal vein

The main adrenal vein is located lying below the adrenal gland and medial to the upper kidney pole. The adrenal vein is then clipped and divided.

Step 5. Completion of adrenal gland mobilisation

The adrenal gland is then fully mobilised using ultrasonic dissection. The final part of the operation is to mobilise the adrenal gland off the peritoneum. If the peritoneum is opened, it does not require subsequent closure.

Step 6. Extraction of the adrenal gland

The adrenal gland is removed through the middle port in an extraction bag. For large adrenal tumours the extraction site can be extended.

Right side

Step 1. Port placement

The camera and instrument ports are placed on the right side using the same technique as the left side.

Step 2. Creation of a retroperitoneal space

A large retroperitoneal space is created using blunt dissection with the laparoscope and blunt dissectors. The adrenal gland tumour and upper pole of the kidney are identified.

Step 3. Initial adrenal gland mobilisation

The upper pole of the kidney is mobilised this allows access to the lower part of the adrenal gland. The adrenal gland is then mobilised laterally around the top of the adrenal gland and continued medially. The adrenal gland arteries were divided by ultrasonic dissection and the posterior surface of the inferior vena cava was identified.

Step 4. Identification and division of main adrenal vein

The inferior vena cava is carefully demonstrated. The short adrenal vein can be seen running postero-laterally. The vein is then clearly identified, clipped and divided.

Step 5. Completion of adrenal gland mobilisation

The fatty tissue between the kidney and adrenal gland are separated. The anterior adhesions between the adrenal gland and peritoneum are separated allowing completion of the mobilisation.

Step 6. Extraction of the adrenal gland

The adrenal gland is removed through the middle port in an extraction bag. For large adrenal tumours the extraction site can be extended.

6.1.4 Uncertainty of laparoscopic adrenalectomy for large (≥6cm) potentially malignant tumours

It is uncertain if the resection of large (≥6cm) potentially malignant adrenal tumours is appropriate due to concern over incomplete resection and local recurrence. However, an increasing number of series have demonstrated the safety of this approach together with low rates of local recurrence. Table 6.2 shows the outcome of studies for the laparoscopic removal of large adrenal tumours.

Author	LA≥6cm over Total LA*	No of patients with malignancy	Tumour size (cm)†	Conversion for large tumours	Incomplete resection	Local recurrence	Mets	Follow-up† (months)
(Henry et al., 2002)	19/233 (8%)	6 (6)	7 (6-8)	2	0	0	1	35 (17-59)
(MacGillivray, Whalen, Malchoff, Oppenheim, & Shichman, 2002)	12/60 (20%)	3 (1)	8 (6-12)	0	0	0	1	24.5 (4-42)
(Walz et al., 2005)	33/429 (8%)	6 (2)	7.3 (2.1)¶	2	n.a.	2	5	n.a.
(Palazzo et al., 2006)	19/391 (5%)	3(3)	6.5 (6-8)	0	n.a.	1	2	25 (13-46)
(Soon et al., 2008)	16/140 (11%)	3 (3)	n.a.	4	n.a.	0	1	18 (n.a.)
(Ramacciato et al., 2008)	20/107ϯ (19%)	4 (2)	8 (7-9)	3	0	0	1	n.a.
Authors series (1999-2009)	69/176 (39%)	20 (10)	8 (6.5-9)	6	0	0	3	41 (22-76)

* Values in parentheses are percentage of LA for tumours ≥6cm or ≥7cm in the case series
ϯ Tumours are 7cm or larger
° Values in parentheses are numbers of primary adrenal cortical carcinomas
† Values are median (IQR) unless stated
¶Value is mean (range)n.a. , data not available

Table 6.2. Laparoscopic adrenalectomy for large adrenal tumours

Currently, we feel like other authors, adopting a policy of LA only for tumours <6cm or highly selecting those with tumours >6cm would prevent a large number of patients receiving the benefits of the laparoscopic approach. Even in the presence of malignancy, laparoscopic resection can achieve very favourable oncological outcomes after long-term follow-up. The laparoscopic approach gives an excellent view of large tumours and radical

resection with a low blood loss can be performed without the need for large abdominal or thoracoabdominal incisions in these patients.
In our series (1999-2009), 69 out of 176 LA were performed for adrenal masses ≥6cm. There were six conversions in this group, mainly for local tumour invasion. Post operative stay for patients with adrenal tumours ≥6cm was a day longer compared to those <6cm (3 days versus 2 days). After a median follow up of 41 months, there has been no clinical or radiological evidence of local recurrence in any patient that has had an attempted laparoscopic approach.

6.2 Laparoscopic subtotal adrenalectomy

Laparoscopic subtotal adrenalectomy has emerged as a feasible option allowing either bilateral adrenal medulla resection or partial adrenal cortex resection in patients with a single remaining adrenal gland (Hardy & Lennard,2008). Case series have reported the procedure is most strongly indicated in patients with bilateral phaeochromocytoma (familial) or patients with aldosterone or cortisol producing tumours who have had previous contralateral adrenalectomy. This has been shown to preserve endogenous steroid production and allow independence from oral steroid therapy in the majority of patients (Brauckhoff et al.,2003).
Selection for subtotal adrenalectomy has generally been performed in small, well circumscribed, peripherally located lesions. It remains unclear from the literature, the true incidence of this procedure as totality of adrenalectomy practice is rarely reported. Results from small studies have reported no incomplete resections or local recurrences (follow-up range:3 months - 3 years) (Walz et al.,1998;Kok&Yapp,2002).

7. Follow-up

7.1 Phaeochromocytomas

Follow-up should be performed indefinitely as the phaeochromocytoma can recur. Follow-up investigations include: urinary catecholamines, CT, MRI and MIBG.

7.2 Adrenocortical carcinoma

For functioning adrenocortical carcinomas, hormonal markers should be measured every 3 months for early detection of tumour recurrence.
Restage by CT (chest, abdomen) every 3-6 months for at least 5 years. This is because recurrent surgical resection is a valid treatment option.

7.3 Conn's syndrome

Following resection, patient is followed up after six weeks. The blood pressure, urea and electrolytes and plasma aldosterone-to-renin ratio are checked. If the results are satisfactory the patients can often be discharged.

7.4 Cushing's syndrome

For patients with Cushing's syndrome (ACTH-independent) resolution of cortisol excess is checked in the postoperative stay. However, the majority of patients remain on steroids and are reviewed in clinic to assess recovery of HPA axis. If this is satisfactory then steroids can be stopped. Postoperative imaging is not usually required.

8. Conclusions

Within an experienced centre (consisting of endocrinologists, anaesthetists and surgeons), laparoscopic adrenalectomy has become the procedure of choice for the vast majority of adrenal pathologies. A large number of case series have consistently demonstrated the improved outcomes of LA compared to the open procedure. We feel, the only contraindications to LA were locally invasive adrenal mass on CT or MRI or the requirement of an additional open surgical procedure. Currently there is no evidence to suggest one laparoscopic approach is better than another. However, the lateral transabdominal approach is currently recommended for adrenal tumours ≥ 6cm.

9. References

Barczynski M, Konturek A, Golkowski F, Cichon S, Huszno B, Peitgen K, Walz MK. (2006). Posterior retroperitoneoscopic adrenalectomy: a comparison between the initial experience in the invention phase and introductory phase of the new surgical technique. World J Surg, 31,65-71.

Boland, G. W., Blake, M. A., Hahn, P. F., & Mayo-Smith, W. W. (2008). Incidental adrenal lesions: Principles, techniques, and algorithms for imaging characterization. *Radiology, 249*(3), 756-775.

Boland, G. W., Lee, M. J., Gazelle, G. S., Halpern, E. F., McNicholas, M. M., & Mueller, P. R. (1998). Characterization of adrenal masses using unenhanced CT: An analysis of the CT literature. *AJR.American Journal of Roentgenology, 171*(1), 201-204.

Bonjer, H. J., Sorm, V., Berends, F. J., Kazemier, G., Steyerberg, E. W., de Herder, W. W., et al. (2000). Endoscopic retroperitoneal adrenalectomy: Lessons learned from 111 consecutive cases. *Annals of Surgery, 232*(6), 796-803.

Bonnet, S., Gaujoux, S., Leconte, M., Thillois, J. M., Tissier, F., & Dousset, B. (2008). Laparoscopic adrenalectomy for metachronous metastasis from renal cell carcinoma. *World Journal of Surgery, 32*(8), 1809-1814.

Bovio, S., Cataldi, A., Reimondo, G., Sperone, P., Novello, S., Berruti, A., et al. (2006). Prevalence of adrenal incidentaloma in a contemporary computerized tomography series. *Journal of Endocrinological Investigation, 29*(4), 298-302.

Brauckhoff, M., Gimm, O., Thanh, P. N., Bar, A., Ukkat, J., Brauckhoff, K., et al. (2003). Critical size of residual adrenal tissue and recovery from impaired early postoperative adrenocortical function after subtotal bilateral adrenalectomy. *Surgery, 134*(6), 1020-1027.

Brauckhoff, M., Stock, K., Stock, S., Lorenz, K., Sekulla, C., Brauckhoff, K., et al. (2008). Limitations of intraoperative adrenal remnant volume measurement in patients undergoing subtotal adrenalectomy. *World Journal of Surgery, 32*(5), 863-872.

Brauckhoff, M., Thanh, P. N., Gimm, O., Bar, A., Brauckhoff, K., & Dralle, H. (2003). Functional results after endoscopic subtotal cortical-sparing adrenalectomy. *Surgery Today, 33*(5), 342-348.

Brunt, L. M., Doherty, G. M., Norton, J. A., Soper, N. J., Quasebarth, M. A., & Moley, J. F. (1996). Laparoscopic adrenalectomy compared to open adrenalectomy for benign adrenal neoplasms. *Journal of the American College of Surgeons, 183*(1), 1-10.

Dudley, N. E., & Harrison, B. J. (1999). Comparison of open posterior versus transperitoneal laparoscopic adrenalectomy. *British Journal of Surgery, 86*(5), 656-660.

Duh, Q. Y. (2002). Adrenal incidentalomas. *British Journal of Surgery, 89*(11), 1347-1349.

Eldeiry, L. S., & Garber, J. R. (2008). Adrenal incidentalomas, 2003 to 2005: Experience after publication of the national institutes of health consensus statement. *Endocrine Practice, 14*(3), 279-284.

Gagner, M., Lacroix, A., & Bolt, E. (1992). Laparoscopic adrenalectomy in cushing's syndrome and pheochromocytoma. *New England Journal of Medicine, the, 327*(14), 1033-1033.

Gagner, M., Pomp, A., Heniford, B. T., Pharand, D., & Lacroix, A. (1997). Laparoscopic adrenalectomy: Lessons learned from 100 consecutive procedures. *Annals of Surgery, 226*(3), 238-246.

Hanssen, W. E., Kuhry, E., Casseres, Y. A., de Herder, W. W., Steyerberg, E. W., & Bonjer, H. J. (2006). Safety and efficacy of endoscopic retroperitoneal adrenalectomy. *British Journal of Surgery, 93*(6), 715-719.

Hardy, R., & Lennard, T. W. (2008). Subtotal adrenalectomy. *British Journal of Surgery, 95*(9), 1075-1076.

Hazzan, D., Shiloni, E., Golijanin, D., Jurim, O., Gross, D., & Reissman, P. (2001). Laparoscopic vs open adrenalectomy for benign adrenal neoplasm. *Surgical Endoscopy, 15*(11), 1356-1358.

Henry, J. F., Sebag, F., Iacobone, M., & Mirallie, E. (2002). Results of laparoscopic adrenalectomy for large and potentially malignant tumors. *World Journal of Surgery, 26*(8), 1043-1047.

Imai, T., Kikumori, T., Ohiwa, M., Mase, T., & Funahashi, H. (1999). A case-controlled study of laparoscopic compared with open lateral adrenalectomy. *American Journal of Surgery, 178*(1), 50-53.

Jacobs, J. K., Goldstein, R. E., & Geer, R. J. (1997). Laparoscopic adrenalectomy. A new standard of care. *Annals of Surgery, 225*(5), 495-501.

Joris, J. L., Hamoir, E. E., Hartstein, G. M., Meurisse, M. R., Hubert, B. M., Charlier, C. J., et al. (1999). Hemodynamic changes and catecholamine release during laparoscopic adrenalectomy for pheochromocytoma. *Anesthesia & Analgesia, 88*(1), 16-21.

Kinney, M. A., Warner, M. E., vanHeerden, J. A., Horlocker, T. T., Young, W. F.,Jr, Schroeder, D. R., et al. (2000). Perianesthetic risks and outcomes of pheochromocytoma and paraganglioma resection. *Anesthesia & Analgesia, 91*(5), 1118-1123.

Kloos, R. T., Gross, M. D., Francis, I. R., Korobkin, M., & Shapiro, B. (1995). Incidentally discovered adrenal masses. *Endocrine Reviews, 16*(4), 460-484.

Kok, K. Y., & Yapp, S. K. (2002). Laparoscopic adrenal-sparing surgery for primary hyperaldosteronism due to aldosterone-producing adenoma. *Surgical Endoscopy, 16*(1), 108-111.

Korobkin, M., Giordano, T. J., Brodeur, F. J., Francis, I. R., Siegelman, E. S., Quint, L. E., et al. (1996). Adrenal adenomas: Relationship between histologic lipid and CT and MR findings. *Radiology, 200*(3), 743-747.

Lebuffe, G., Dosseh, E. D., Tek, G., Tytgat, H., Moreno, S., Tavernier, B., et al. (2005). The effect of calcium channel blockers on outcome following the surgical treatment of phaeochromocytomas and paragangliomas. *Anaesthesia, 60*(5), 439-444.

Lee, J. E., Evans, D. B., Hickey, R. C., Sherman, S. I., Gagel, R. F., Abbruzzese, M. C., et al. (1998). Unknown primary cancer presenting as an adrenal mass: Frequency and implications for diagnostic evaluation of adrenal incidentalomas. *Surgery, 124*(6), 1115-1122.

Linos, D. A., Stylopoulos, N., Boukis, M., Souvatzoglou, A., Raptis, S., & Papadimitriou, J. (1997). Anterior, posterior, or laparoscopic approach for the management of adrenal diseases?. *American Journal of Surgery, 173*(2), 120-125.

MacGillivray, D. C., Shichman, S. J., Ferrer, F. A., & Malchoff, C. D. (1996). A comparison of open vs laparoscopic adrenalectomy. *Surgical Endoscopy, 10*(10), 987-990.

MacGillivray, D. C., Whalen, G. F., Malchoff, C. D., Oppenheim, D. S., & Shichman, S. J. (2002). Laparoscopic resection of large adrenal tumors. *Annals of Surgical Oncology, 9*(5), 480-485.

Mercan, S., Seven, R., Ozarmagan, S., & Tezelman, S. (1995). Endoscopic retroperitoneal adrenalectomy. *Surgery, 118*(6), 1071-1075.

Nieman LK. (2010). Approach to the patient with an adrenal incidentaloma. J Clin Endocrinol Metab, 95(9), 4106-4113.

Ortega, J., Sala, C., Garcia, S., & Lledo, S. (2002). Cost-effectiveness of laparoscopic vs open adrenalectomy: Small savings in an expensive process. *Journal of Laparoendoscopic & Advanced Surgical Techniques.Part A, 12*(1), 1-5.

Palazzo, F. F., Sebag, F., Sierra, M., Ippolito, G., Souteyrand, P., & Henry, J. F. (2006). Long-term outcome following laparoscopic adrenalectomy for large solid adrenal cortex tumors. *World Journal of Surgery, 30*(5), 893-898.

Park, B. K., Kim, C. K., Kim, B., & Lee, J. H. (2007). Comparison of delayed enhanced CT and chemical shift MR for evaluating hyperattenuating incidental adrenal masses. *Radiology, 243*(3), 760-765.

Plouin, P. F., Duclos, J. M., Soppelsa, F., Boublil, G., & Chatellier, G. (2001). Factors associated with perioperative morbidity and mortality in patients with pheochromocytoma: Analysis of 165 operations at a single center. *Journal of Clinical Endocrinology & Metabolism, 86*(4), 1480-1486.

Prys-Roberts, C. (2000). Phaeochromocytoma--recent progress in its management. *British Journal of Anaesthesia, 85*(1), 44-57.

Prys-Roberts, C., & Farndon, J. R. (2002). Efficacy and safety of doxazosin for perioperative management of patients with pheochromocytoma. *World Journal of Surgery, 26*(8), 1037-1042.

Ramacciato, G., Mercantini, P., La Torre, M., Di Benedetto, F., Ercolani, G., Ravaioli, M., et al. (2008). Is laparoscopic adrenalectomy safe and effective for adrenal masses larger than 7 cm?. *Surgical Endoscopy, 22*(2), 516-521.

Rayan, S. S., & Hodin, R. A. (2000). Short-stay laparoscopic adrenalectomy. *Surgical Endoscopy, 14*(6), 568-572.

Ross, E. J., Prichard, B. N., Kaufman, L., Robertson, A. I., & Harries, B. J. (1967). Preoperative and operative management of patients with phaeochromocytoma. *British Medical Journal, 1*(5534), 191-198.

Sasano, H., Shizawa, S., & Nagura, H. (1995). Adrenocortical cytopathology. *American Journal of Clinical Pathology, 104*(2), 161-166.

Saunders, B. D., Wainess, R. M., Dimick, J. B., Upchurch, G. R., Doherty, G. M., & Gauger, P. G. (2004). Trends in utilization of adrenalectomy in the united states: Have indications changed?. *World Journal of Surgery, 28*(11), 1169-1175.

Schell, S. R., Talamini, M. A., & Udelsman, R. (1999). Laparoscopic adrenalectomy for nonmalignant disease: Improved safety, morbidity, and cost-effectiveness. *Surgical Endoscopy, 13*(1), 30-34.

Shen, W. T., Lim, R. C., Siperstein, A. E., Clark, O. H., Schecter, W. P., Hunt, T. K., et al. (1999). Laparoscopic vs open adrenalectomy for the treatment of primary hyperaldosteronism. *Archives of Surgery, 134*(6), 628-631.

Soares, R. L.,Jr, Monchik, J., Migliori, S. J., & Amaral, J. F. (1999). Laparoscopic adrenalectomy for benign adrenal neoplasms. *Surgical Endoscopy, 13*(1), 40-42.

Song, J. H., Chaudhry, F. S., & Mayo-Smith, W. W. (2007). The incidental indeterminate adrenal mass on CT (> 10 H) in patients without cancer: Is further imaging necessary? follow-up of 321 consecutive indeterminate adrenal masses. *AJR.American Journal of Roentgenology, 189*(5), 1119-1123.

Soon, P. S., Yeh, M. W., Delbridge, L. W., Bambach, C. P., Sywak, M. S., Robinson, B. G., et al. (2008). Laparoscopic surgery is safe for large adrenal lesions. *European Journal of Surgical Oncology, 34*(1), 67-70.

Staren, E. D., & Prinz, R. A. (1996). Adrenalectomy in the era of laparoscopy. *Surgery, 120*(4), 706-709.

Sturgeon, C., Shen, W. T., Clark, O. H., Duh, Q. Y., & Kebebew, E. (2006). Risk assessment in 457 adrenal cortical carcinomas: How much does tumor size predict the likelihood of malignancy?. *Journal of the American College of Surgeons, 202*(3), 423-430.

Tauzin-Fin, P., Sesay, M., Gosse, P., & Ballanger, P. (2004). Effects of perioperative alpha1 block on haemodynamic control during laparoscopic surgery for phaeochromocytoma. *British Journal of Anaesthesia, 92*(4), 512-517.

Thompson, G. B., Grant, C. S., van Heerden, J. A., Schlinkert, R. T., Young, W. F.,Jr, Farley, D. R., et al. (1997). Laparoscopic versus open posterior adrenalectomy: A case-control study of 100 patients. *Surgery, 122*(6), 1132-1136.

Thompson, G. B., & Young, W. F.,Jr. (2003). Adrenal incidentaloma. *Current Opinion in Oncology, 15*(1), 84-90.

Ting, A. C., Lo, C. Y., & Lo, C. M. (1998). Posterior or laparoscopic approach for adrenalectomy. *American Journal of Surgery, 175*(6), 488-490.

Vargas, H. I., Kavoussi, L. R., Bartlett, D. L., Wagner, J. R., Venzon, D. J., Fraker, D. L., et al. (1997). Laparoscopic adrenalectomy: A new standard of care. *Urology, 49*(5), 673-678.

Walz, M. K., Alesina, P. F., Wenger, F. A., Deligiannis, A., Szuczik, E., Petersenn, S., et al. (2006). Posterior retroperitoneoscopic adrenalectomy--results of 560 procedures in 520 patients. *Surgery, 140*(6), 943-948.

Walz, M. K., Peitgen, K., Saller, B., Giebler, R. M., Lederbogen, S., Nimtz, K., et al. (1998). Subtotal adrenalectomy by the posterior retroperitoneoscopic approach. *World Journal of Surgery, 22*(6), 621-626.

Walz, M. K., Petersenn, S., Koch, J. A., Mann, K., Neumann, H. P., & Schmid, K. W. (2005). Endoscopic treatment of large primary adrenal tumours. *British Journal of Surgery, 92*(6), 719-723.

Winfield, H. N., Hamilton, B. D., Bravo, E. L., & Novick, A. C. (1998). Laparoscopic adrenalectomy: The preferred choice? A comparison to open adrenalectomy. *Journal of Urology, 160*(2), 325-329.

Young, W. F.,Jr. (2000). Management approaches to adrenal incidentalomas. A view from rochester, minnesota. *Endocrinology & Metabolism Clinics of North America, 29*(1), 159-185.

9

Laparoscopic Hernia Repair and Its Validation by Second-Look Inspection to Internal Inguinal Rings in Children with Patent Processus Vaginalis

Masao Endo, Michinobu Ohno, Fumiko Yoshida,
Miwako Nakano, Toshihiko Watanabe and Etsuji Ukiyama
Department of Pediatric Surgery, Saitama City Hospital
Japan

1. Introduction

We developed a unique technique for achieving the completely extraperitoneal ligation of a patent processus vaginalis (PPV) without skipping any areas (Endo et al., 2001). This technique has been used for the treatment of more than 1,600 children. A previous comparative study of this technique with the traditional cut-down repair method proved the superiority of this technique with respect to the parental perspective and choice, operative time, recurrence rate, metachronous appearance of contralateral hernia, complication of the reproductive system, and cosmetic results (Endo et al., 2009).
However, some concerns have been voiced regarding the use of laparoscopic herniorrhaphy in children such as the use of a simple closure without the division of the hernial sac, evidence of a completely closed internal inguinal ring (IIR), validity with regard to future recurrence, and the high risk of adhesion (Miltenburg et al., 1998, Gorsler et al., 2003, Saranga et al., 2008).
Since 1996, when we began to close PPV laparoscopically, we have conducted prospective studies involving laparoscopic inspection at previous operation sites at every opportunity so as to validate the efficacy of this procedure. The purpose of this paper was to introduce our procedure and the use of recently devised, innovative "Endoneedle kit", comparing the outcome, including the morphological appearance of the IIRs in second-look operations, with the outcome of traditional cut-down herniorrhaphy performed during the same period.

2. Materials and methods

[Operative procedures] The kit consists of a 70 mm needle covered with a 17-G metal sheath (puncture needle), an 18-G dull-tipped needle with a wire loop inside the barrel for the internal introduction of a 2-0 suture used to send the suture (suture sender), and a 20-G dull-tipped needle with a wire loop inside the barrel used to retrieve the suture (suture retriever)(Fig.1). These needles are packaged together and provided as a sterilized, non-reusable package.

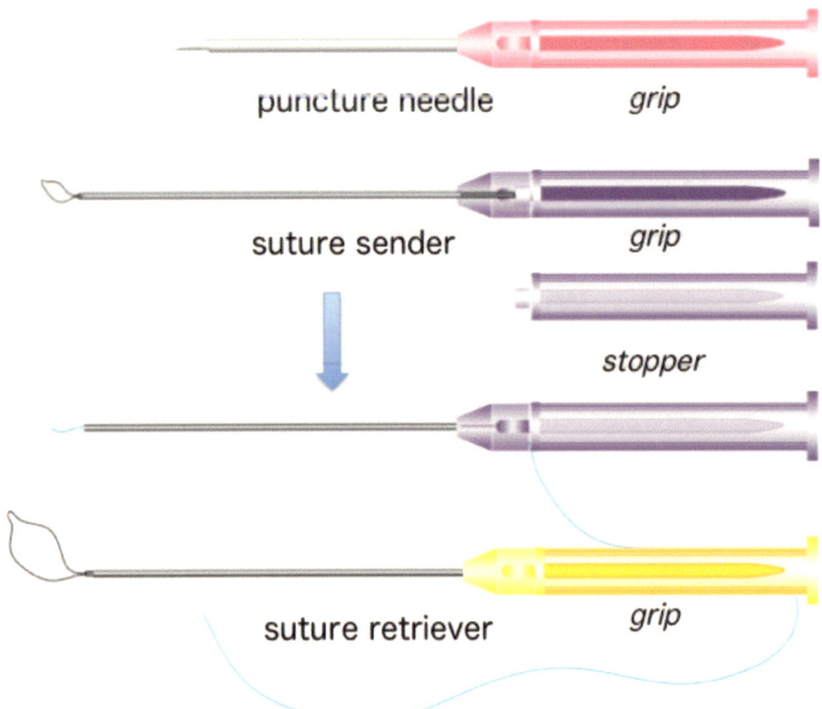

Fig. 1. Composition of the Endoneedle Kit. The needle contained inside the puncture needle can be released by twisting and pulling the grip. The suture (0-2 non-absorbable twisted suture) is pulled through the barrel of the suture sender and fixed with a stopper. The suture is picked up by a grasper through the loop of the suture retriever and caught by pulling back the grip.

The puncture needle is inserted percutaneously and advanced along the lower half of the IIR extraperitoneally across the cord and vessels and protruded into the peritoneal space at the opposite side of the puncture site, then withdrawn leaving the metal sheath in place. A 2-0 suture is then delivered into the peritoneal space through the metal sheath using the suture sender and placed at the site by withdrawing the sheath and the suture sender. The puncture needle is then advanced along the upper half of the IIR and protruded into the peritoneal space at the site where the previously sent suture has penetrated the peritoneum. The suture is then retrieved by the suture retriever passed through the metal sheath of the puncture needle and tied extracorporeally, enabling a complete extraperitoneal ligation of the ring (Fig.2).

[Study design] A consecutive series of 1,943 children who underwent definitive herniorrhaphy between 1996 and 2009 was analyzed. At the preoperative guidance session, three methods were proposed to the patients' parents (Fig.3): a traditional cut-down repair (CDR) for the affected side only (CDR-A), an additional diagnostic laparoscopy for contralateral IIR inspection with simultaneous closure of the contralateral PPV (cPPV) (CDR+L), and a laparoscopic completely extraperitoneal PPV closure with routine closure of the cPPV during the same procedure (LCEPC). Either a CDR-A, CDR+L or LCEPC was selected according to the parent's preference and with their informed consent.

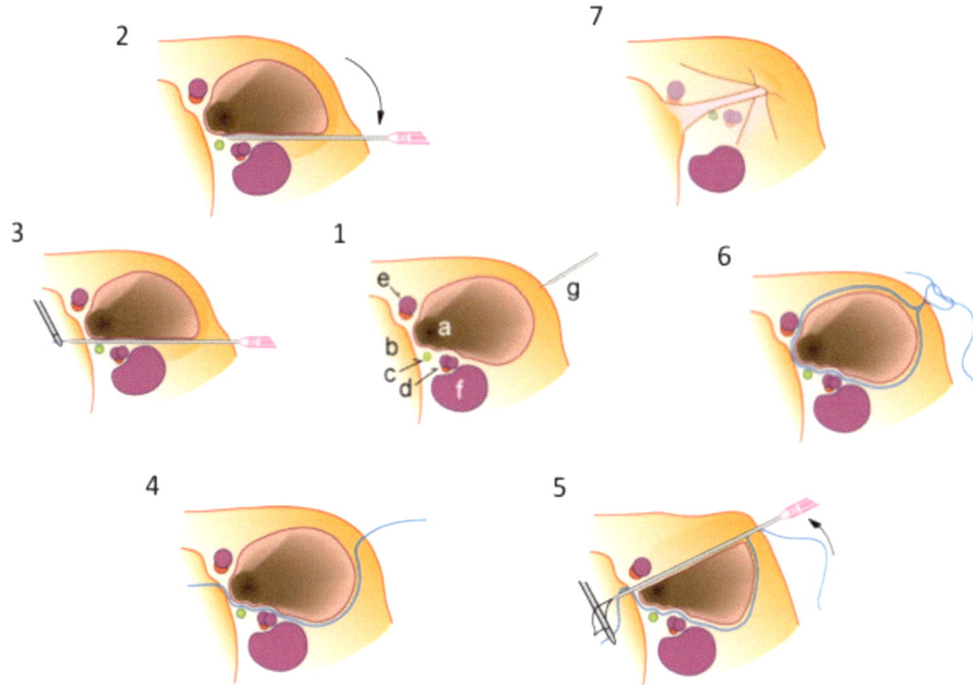

Fig. 2. Schematic drawing of completely extraperitoneal closure of the right-sided PPV. 1. Anatomy of male IIR. a, orifice of PPV; b, wall of pelvic pouch; c, spermatic duct; d, testicular vessels; e, inferior epigastric vessels; f, external iliac vein, g, puncture needle being inserted percutaneously. 2. The puncture needle goes extraperitoneally across the common iliac vein, testicular vessels and spermatic cord, which are easily facilitated by pressing the needle down. 3. A suture is carried into the peritoneal cavity by the suture sender and picked up by a grasper. 4. The suture is left along the lower half of the IIR. 5. The free end of the suture is picked up by the suture retriever inserted through the puncture needle that has been placed along the upper half of the IIR. 6. The orifice of the PPV has been encircled without any skip area. 7. The IIR has been tied up, while the spermatic cord and the testicular vessels are drawn close to the ligation but spared.

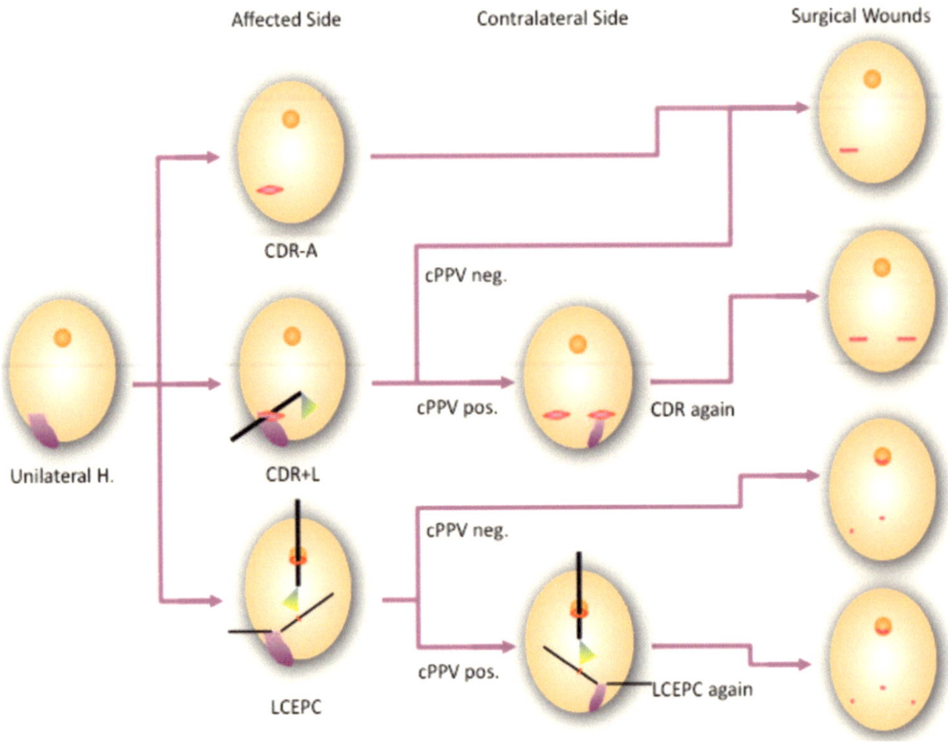

Fig. 3. Instruction for parental perspective and choice. There are three choices; 1, cut-down repair for affected side only (CDR-A); 2, CDR with diagnostic laparoscopy with CDR again for cPPV if present (CDR+L); 3, laparoscopic completely extraperitoneal PPV closure with simultaneous closure for cPPV (LCEPC).

The LCEPC and CDR groups were then compared according to parental selection, distribution of sex, age, clinical lateralities, associated morbidities, operation times, development of contralateral hernia, recurrence and major complications. The patients were followed up regularly in our outpatient clinic for 7 months after the operation, and during visits for any other complaints or morbidities thereafter. The follow-up period ranged from one to 14 years.

Among these children, the IIRs of 58 children who had undergone a second laparoscopic operation were investigated with regard to the morphological appearance of the IIRs during the revisit, with special reference to the predicted future outcome. The distributions of the primary operations of these 58 children and the reasons for the second operation are showed in Figure 4.

Based on the procedure used for the primary operation, the IIRs were classified into a post-cut-down repair group (post-CDR) and a post-laparoscopic repair group (post-LCEPC). Among the IIRs that were inspected, those found to be closed (closed IIR = C-IIR) were investigated in terms of their morphological variations: from a flat scar to degeneration with a dimple, cicatricial tissue gathering, or adhesion. The spectra of the morphological deviations were compared between the post-CDR and post-LCEPC groups.

[Statistical analysis] Continuous data were expressed as the mean +/- standard deviation (SD). Statistical significance was calculated using a two-tailed *t*-test. For proportional data, the chi-square test was used.

3. Results

[Results for definitive herniorrhaphy]

Parents showed a greater preference for LCEPC, accounting for 1,631 children (86%) compared with 312 children who underwent CDR with or without a diagnostic laparoscopy (CDR-A, 66; CDR+L, 246) (Fig. 5).

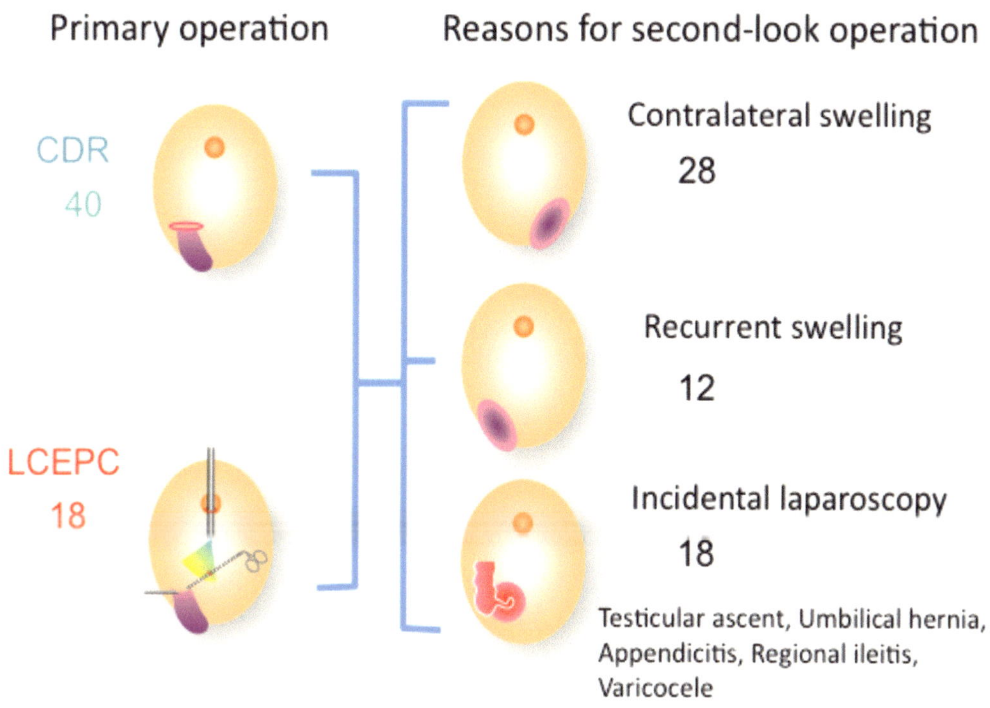

Fig. 4. Distributions of primary operation and reasons for second-look operation. Incidental laparoscopies were performed during treatment for testicular ascent (8), umbilical hernia (4), appendicitis (2), regional ileitis (1), varicocele (1) and miscellaneous (2). Numbers in parenthesis indicate numbers of patient.

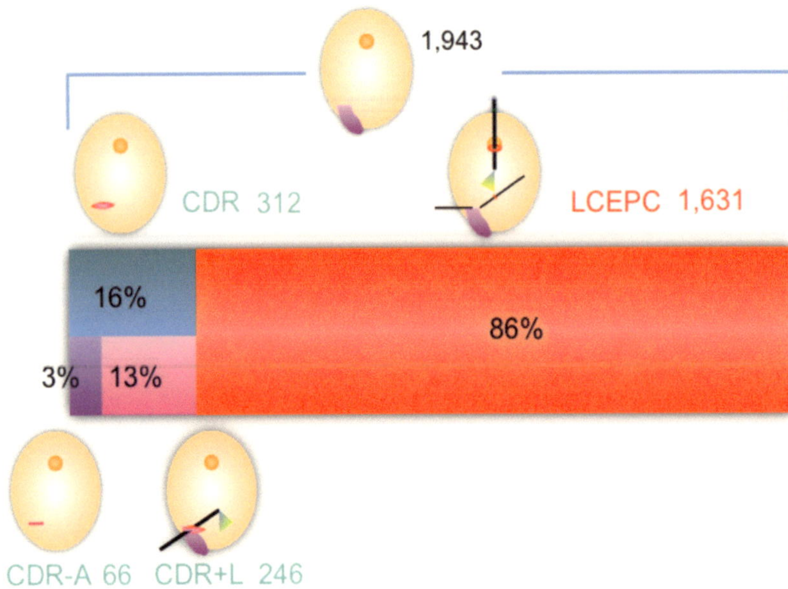

Fig. 5. Patients who underwent chosen procedures. Total number of patients was 1,943; Number of patients in LCEPC group was 1,631 (86%) and in CDR was 312 (16%), in which CDR-A was 66 (3%) and CDR+L was 246 (13%).

The age distributions for the CDR and LCEPC groups (around 3.9 and 3.7 years, respectively) were not significantly different (Fig. 6).

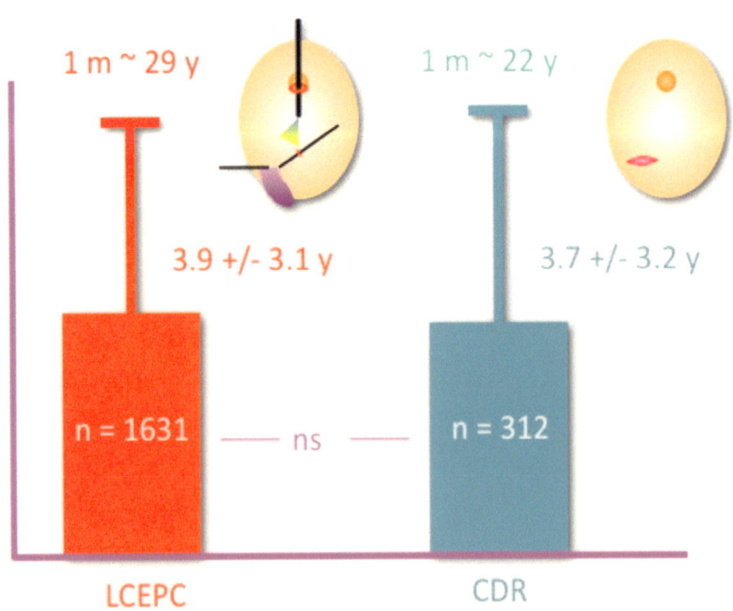

Fig. 6. Distribution of ages. Data are shown in mean +/- standard deviation. ns, statistically not significant.

The distribution of clinical hernia sides was also the same for both groups (Fig. 7).

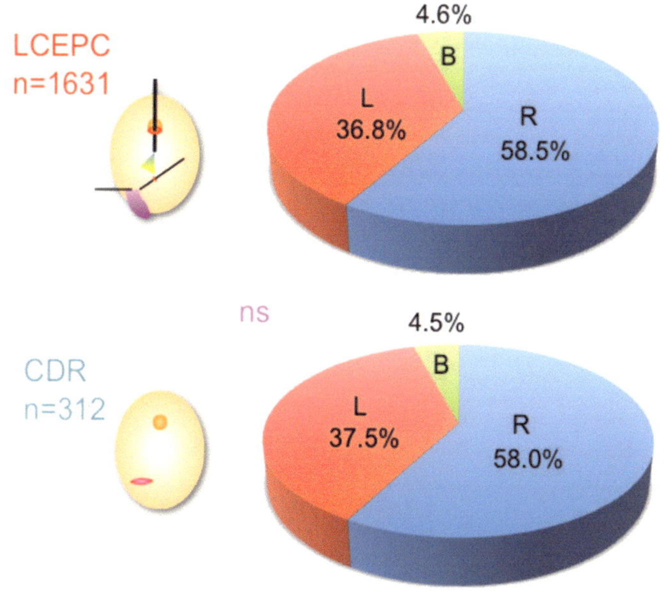

Fig. 7. Distributions of lateralities in clinical hernia. Differences between both groups were not statistically significant.

On the other hand, the sex distribution showed a female predominance in the LCEPC group because of the parents' perspective regarding the cosmetic superiority of laparoscopic repair (Fig. 8).

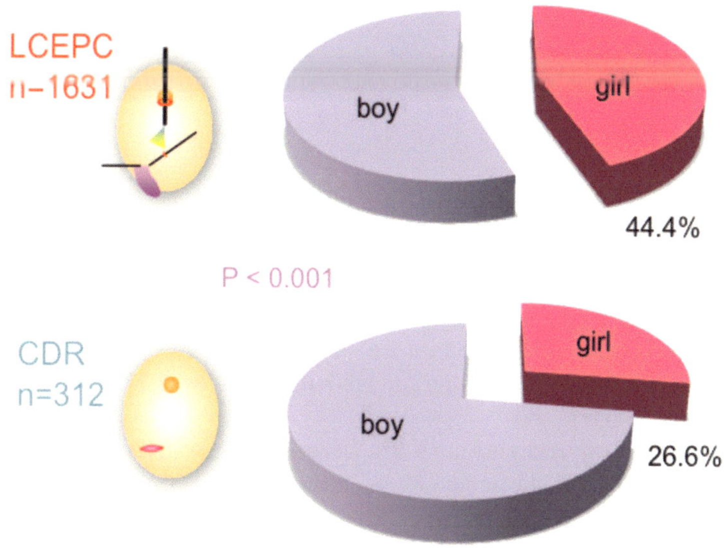

Fig. 8. Sex distribution. LCEPC group included more girls (44.4%) than CDR group (26.6%), $p<0.001$.

Regarding the distributions of associated morbidities necessitating a combined operation, no statistically significant differences were observed between the two groups with the exception of umbilical hernia/cysts. Umbilical deformities were seen 4 times more frequently in the LCEPC group because of the parental desire for an umbilicoplasty during the same session (Fig. 9).

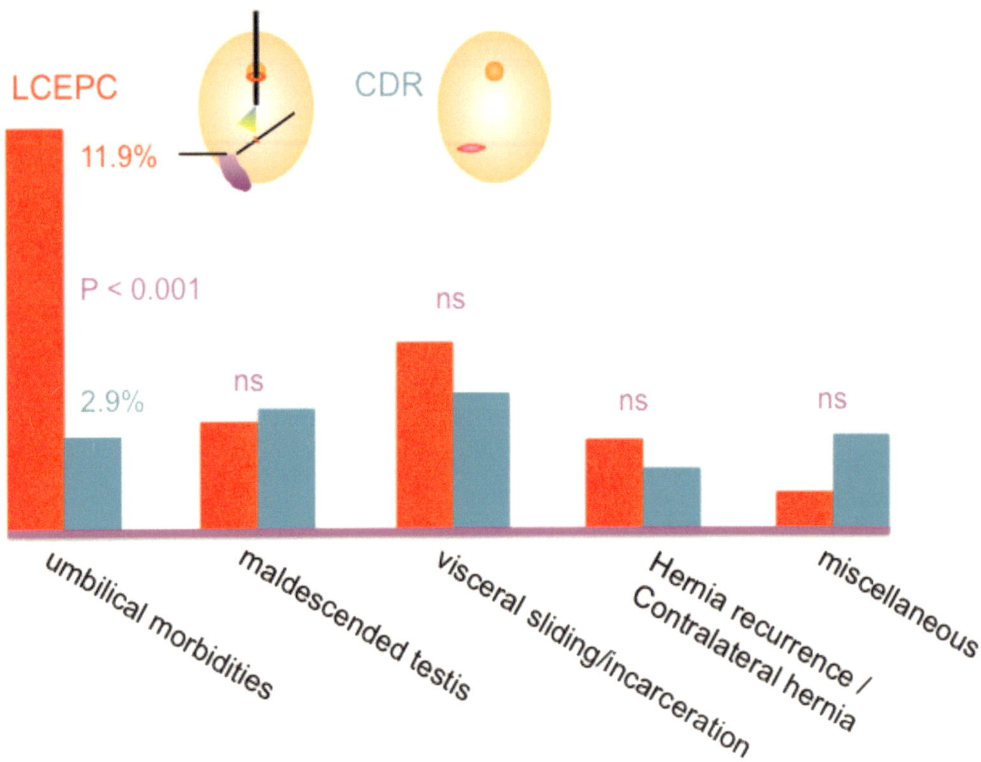

Fig. 9. Associated morbidities necessitating a combined operation. There were no statistically significant differences in the distributions of associated morbidities except umbilical morbidities such as hernia, cystic degeneration or ugly-looking umbilicus (LCEPC, 194, 11.9% vs. CDR, 9, 2.9%, $p<0.001$).

The mean operation times for unilateral repair were the same in the LCEPC and CDR groups, while the mean operation time for bilateral repair was 11 minutes shorter in the LCEPC group ($p<0.001$) (Fig. 10).

Intra- and post-operative complications are listed in Table 1. A statistically significant difference was observed in the incidence of intra-operative injuries to the reproductive system between the LCEPC and CDR groups (0% vs. 0.6%, $p<0,001$). The incidence of postoperative contralateral hernia was lower in the LCEPC group, but the difference was not statistically significant. Postoperative hernia recurrence was significantly lower in the LCEPC group ($p<0.001$).

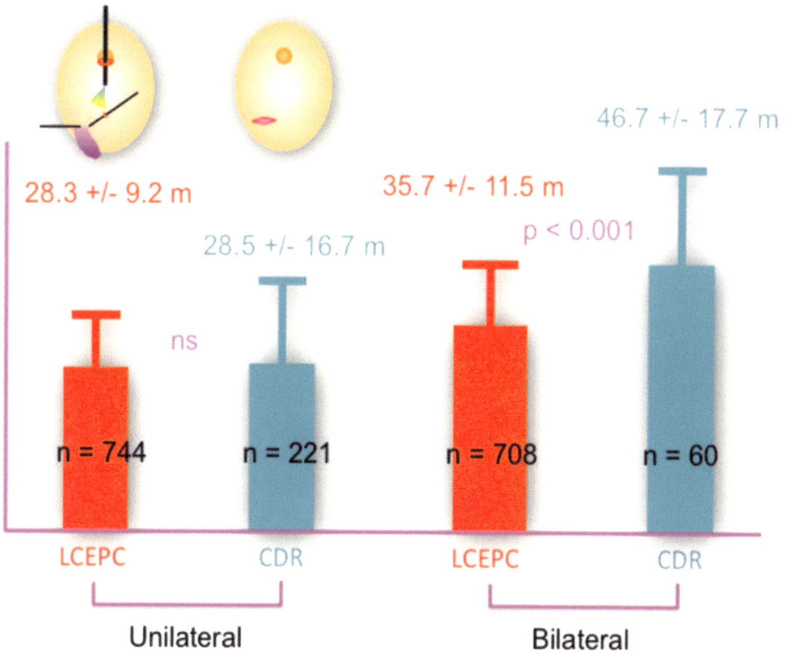

Fig. 10. Operation times in LCEPC and CDR groups. Operation times for unilateral repair were equal in both LCEPC and CDR groups (28.3 +/- 9.2 m for LCEPC vs. 28.5 +/- 16.7 m for CDR) and were shorter for LCEPC group in bilateral repair (35.7 +/- 11.5 m vs. 46.7 +/- 17.7 m, p<0.001). Patients who underwent combined operations affecting definitive herniorrhaphy were excluded from the analysis.

	LCEPC	CDR	Difference
Major complication*	0/1631 pts 0.00%	2/312 pts 0.64%	P<0.001
Contralateral hernia	5/814 UCs 0.61%	4/246 UCs 1.63%	n.s.
Hernia recurrence	2/1631 pts 0.12%	3/312 pts 0.96%	P<0.001
	2/2428 PPVs 0.08%	3/378 PPVs 0.79%	P<0.001

Table 1. Intraoperative and postoperative complications. Abbreviations: pts, patients; UCs, unilateral closures; n.s., not significant; PPVs, patent processus vaginalis; *, injury to ovarian duct and spermatic duct in a patient, respectively.

[Results for second-look operations]

Among the 58 children, a total of 97 IIRs were investigated, including 36 C-IIRs in the post-CDR group and 23 C-IIRs in the post-LCEPC group. The C-IIRs were classified according to the morphological findings during the operation, as follows: flat type, in which the IIR was flat and covered with thin cicatricial tissue; dimpled type, in which the IIR was covered by a dimpled scar; convergence type, in which cicatricial tissue had gathered at the center of the closed IIR; adhesion type, in which the IIR had adhesive bands from the surrounding viscera; convex type, in which the IIR bulged into the peritoneal cavity with a thick scar formation; and rod type, in which the IIR showed the rod-like protrusion of a thick scar (Fig. 11).

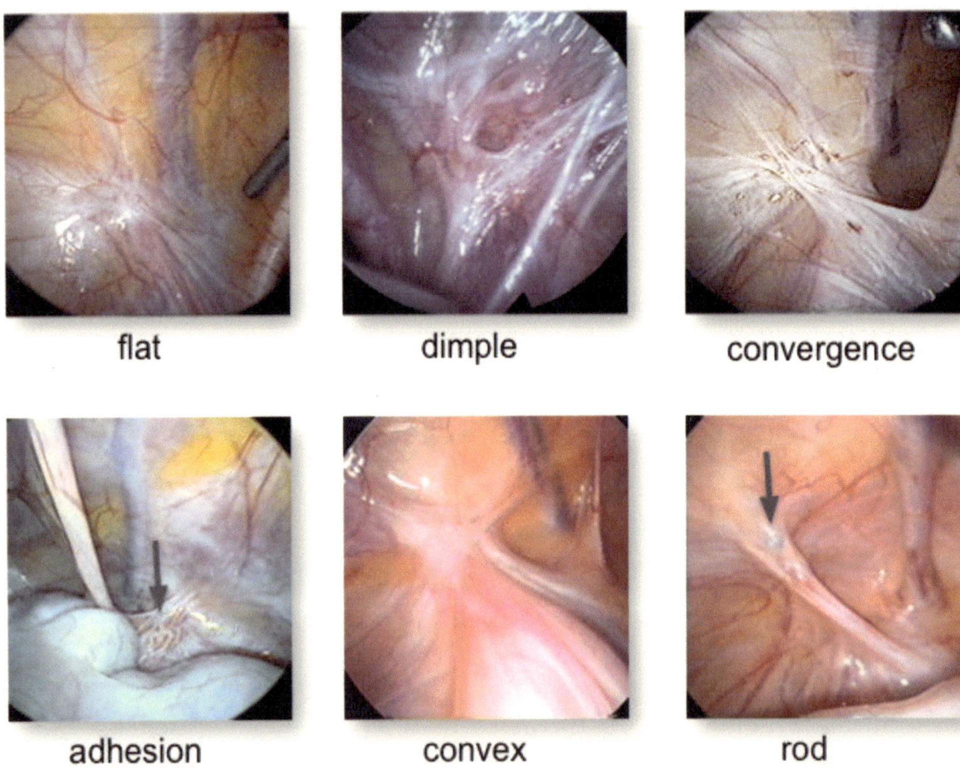

Fig. 11. Spectrum of the morphological findings of closed IIRs. Type "flat", IIR is covered with thin cicatricial tissue resembling congenitally obliterated IIR; type "dimple", IIR has thick cicatricial tissue and a dimple at the center looks like recurrence of the PPV; type "convergence", thick cicatricial tissues are gathering in the center of depressed IIR; type "adhesion", adhesive bands are seen from surrounding viscera (cecum in this example) and dislocated sutures are also seen in some cases (arrow); type "convex", IIR is covered with thick scar tissue and convex toward the intraperitoneal space; type "rod", IIR has a rod like thickening of the scar tissue protruding into the peritoneal cavity. A suture knot is seen at the closure site in this case (arrow).

The C-IIRs in the post-CDR group were mostly composed of the flat type, followed in frequency by the dimpled, convergence and adhesion types indicating that most of the closed IIRs were of the flat or dimpled type with/without peritoneal convergence or adhesions. On the other hand, the C-IIRs in the post-LCEPC group mostly consisted of the flat, rod or convex types, with only one case with a dimpled type, indicating that 95.7% of the closed IIRs were of a flat or convex type bulging into the peritoneal space (Fig. 12). This difference in the distribution of morphological findings was significantly different between the two groups (p<0.001).

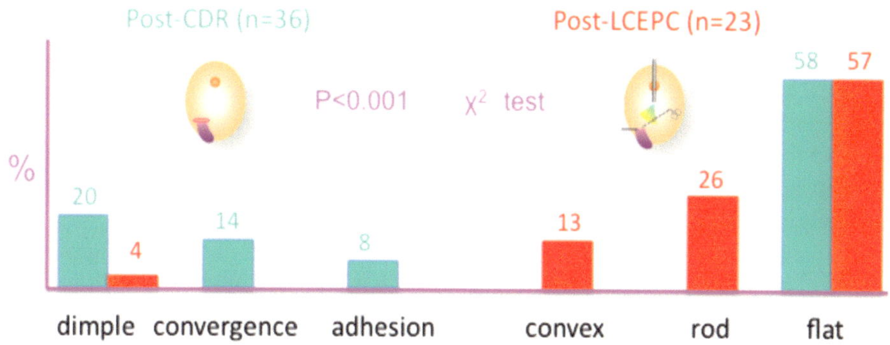

Fig. 12. Distribution of morphological appearances of the closed IIR. More than half IIRs in both groups revealed type "flat". In remaining cases, IIRs in CDR group showed types having any degenerative changes such as "dimple", "convergence" or "adhesion", while IIRs in LCEPC group had types looking like a solid foundation such as "convex" or "rod". Differences between two groups was statistically significant, p<0.001.

4. Discussion

When we reported our initial experience with our technique for the laparoscopic repair of indirect inguinal hernias, some concerns existed regarding the procedure. What is the advantage of laparoscopic herniorrhaphy in children? Is it tolerable to increase the intra-abdominal pressure, despite the simple closure without dividing the hernial sac? Is there any evidence that the IIR is completely closed? How can the improbability of future recurrence and the risk of adhesion be validated? Despite these questions, the primary operation sites between cases that had undergone traditional open surgery and those that have undergone laparoscopic herniorrhaphy have not been previously compared in terms of long-term outcome.

The aim of our project was based on the principle of the traditional cut-down technique involving complete extraperitoneal high ligation of the PPV and to minimize the above concerns by using a simple technique. We devised a set of needles to enable a complete circumferential ligation of the PPV using a suture that is delivered percutaneously via an extraperitoneal route in a manner that is both easy to perform and safe. The needle passes beneath the ligamentum teres uteri distal to the U-turned ovarian duct in girls, involving the ligament inside the ligature. To avoid damage to the spermatic cord and testicular vessels in boys, the needle is advanced between the peritoneum, and the cord and vessels.

At the beginning of the trial, we used some equipment that was available at that time, such as a Deschamps' needle or a biopsy needle. The key point of this technique is to pass a suture in and out around the IIR percutaneously under safe conditions and with precise control. After several modifications, we developed a commercial product that we named the "Endoneedle Kit". This kit can be easily used with satisfactory results and provides precise control while reducing the operation time.

Regarding the parents' perspective, the parents chose laparoscopic repair more frequently because they highly valued the cPPV closure and the cosmetic superiority, resulting in the predominance of girls and the associated morbidities of the umbilicus in the LCEPC group. The parents were very satisfied with the wound and umbilical cosmesis in the LCEPC group patients.

The average operation time for a unilateral hernia in the LCEPC group was comparable with that in the CDR group but was shorter for bilateral hernias. The technology was much easier to use in girls than in boys, as care is required around the spermatic cord. Because of the tight contact between the spermatic cord and the peritoneum, the separation of these structures in advance using electrocautery and a grasper is advisable (Endo et al., 2009), although in skilled hands, this step can be abridged.

Drawbacks associated with the reproductive system are a hidden but not negligible problem (Steigman et al., 1999, Hansen et al., 2006). We had two episodes of injury to the reproductive system during cut-down repair. On the other hand, direct intraoperative inspection of the spermatic cord and/or adnexa enables injury to these structures to be avoided.

As for postoperative complications, the incidence of metachronous hernia among children who underwent LCEPC was 0.6%, which was far lower than reported incidence for traditional unilateral open repair (between 5.6% and 30%)(Given et al., 1989, Burd et al., 2001). Postoperative recurrence was significantly less frequent in the LCEPC group. The main factors affecting recurrence have been recognized as (1) failure to ligate the sac high enough at the internal ring, (2) injury to the floor of the inguinal canal as a result of operative trauma, (3) failure to close the internal ring in girls, and (4) postoperative wound infection and hematoma (Grosfeld et al., 1991). Our technique has proven to be a method that can avoid all these possible causes of recurrence.

To further validate the efficacy of laparoscopic closure of the PPV with regard to postoperative complications, we analyzed the laparoscopically inspected IIRs that had been closed with a definitive herniorrhaphy. A laparoscopic approach during a second-look operation enabled the correct relationships of the anatomic structures to be identified under direct vision.

Laparoscopically observed C-IIRs varied widely in appearance, ranging from a flat closed ring with scarring to somewhat protruded or depressed rings with or without cicatricial gathering, and with or without adhesive bands from the surrounding viscera. In both the post-CDR and post-LCEPC groups, approximately 50% of the children exhibited a flat closed ring without cicatricial gathering or adhesion, which was thought to indicate the unlikelihood of problems in the future. In the remaining 50%, however, characteristic differences were found in the spectra of variations between the post-CDR and post-LCEPC groups. Most of the C-IIRs in the post-CDR group were of the flat or depressed type, while some showed cicatricial gathering or adhesions from the bladder, cecum or the omentum. In contrast, the C-IIRs in the post-LCEPC group ranged from flat to convex or the rod-like convexity type without cicatricial gathering or adhesions. This difference may have arisen from the difference in the approach to the IIR. In laparoscopic closure, the IIR is encircled by a suture proximal to the IIR level, placing all the surrounding viscera out of the IIR, while the cut-down procedure requires the traction of the seminal cord or round ligament from the outside so as to obtain a good visual field and achieve high ligation. The omental or intestinal loop protrusion into the operative field during closure is a common experience when the intraabdominal pressure rises because of inadequate anesthesia. A flat or convex type of IIR without any adhesions, as observed in the post-LCEPC group, may enable the maintenance of an anatomically normal IIR structure over the long-term.

5. Conclusion

We reported the unique technique to achieve completely extraperitoneal ligation of the PPV without any skip areas, sparing the spermatic cord and vessels under laparoscopic control, investigating the outcome, including the morphological appearance of the IIRs during second-look operations, with the outcome of traditional cut-down herniorrhaphy performed during the same period. Our technique as several advantages: the technique is easy to perform and requires a short operation time, it enables the inspection of bilateral IIRs with simultaneous closure of the cPPV, it is associated with a minimum incidence of hernia recurrence and contralateral hernia, the reproductive systems can be left intact, the routine addition of an umbilicoplasty can be performed as needed, and the resulting wound is essentially indiscernible. The present comparative study, which included a second-look investigation of the IIRs, validated the feasibility of laparoscopic closure of the PPV, suggesting that this technique should be regarded as the gold standard for the treatment of children with an indirect inguinal hernia.

6. Acknowledgments

The authors gratefully acknowledge the cooperation of TSK Laboratory, Japan for developing this "Endoneedle Kit".

7. References

[1] Burd RS., Heffington SH., & Teague JL. (2001), The optimal approach for management of metachronous hernias in children: a decision analysis. *J Pediatr Surg*, 36:1190-1995

[2] Endo M., & Ukiyama E. (2001). Laparoscopic closure of patent processus vaginalis in girls with inguinal hernia using a specially devised suture needle. *Ped Endosurg Innov Techn* 5(2):187-191, 1092-6410

[3] Endo M., Watanabe T., Nakano M., Yoshida F., & Ukiyama E (2009), Laparoscopic completely extraperitoneal repair of inguinal hernia in children: A single institute experience with 1,257 repairs compared with cut-down herniorrhaphy. *Surg Endosc*, 23(8):1706-1712.

[4] Given JP., & Rubin SZ. (1989), Occurrence of contralateral inguinal hernia following unilateral repair in a pediatric hospital. *J Pediatr Surg*, 24:963-965

[5] Gorsler CM., & Schier F. (2003), Laparoscopic herniorrhaphy in children. *Surg Endosc*, 17(4):571-573

[6] Grosfeld JL., Minnick K., Shedd F., West KW., Rescoria FJ., & Vane DW. (1991), Inguinal hernia in children: factors affecting recurrence in 62 cases. *J Pediatr Surg*, 26:283-287

[7] Hansen KA., & Eyster KM. (2006), Infertility: an unusual complication of inguinal herniorrhaphy. *Fertil Steril*, 86:217-218

[8] Miltenburg DM., Nuchtern JG., Jaksic T., Kozinetiz C., & Brandt ML. (1998), Laparoscopic evaluation of the pediatric hernia- A meta-analysis. *J Pediatr Surg,* 33(6):874-879

[9] Saranga BR., Arora M., & Baskaran V. (2008), Pediatric inguinal hernia: laparoscopic versus open surgery. *JSLS,* 12(3): 277-281.

[10] Steigman CK., Sotelo-Avila C., & Weber TR. (1999), The incidence of spermatic cord structures in inguinal hernia sacs from male children. *Am J Surg Pathol,* 23: 880-885